C000171423

Tess Connors

PALEO DIET

FOR WOMEN

NEW PALEO RECIPES TO LOSE WEIGHT,
REDUCE CELLULITE AND HAVE MORE ENERGY

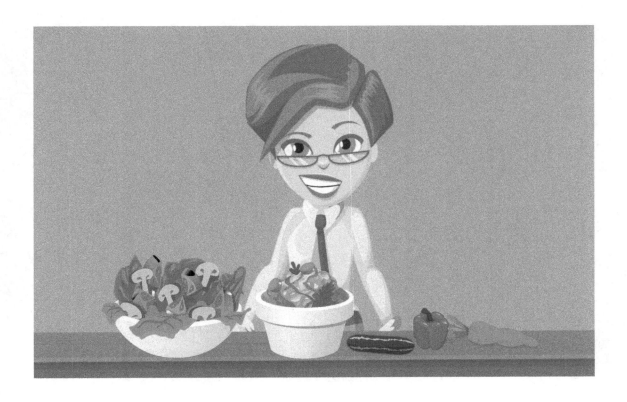

Copyright 2021 – All rights reserved.

The content contained within this book may not be reproduced, duplicated or transmitted without direct written permission from the author or the publisher.

Under no circumstances will any blame or legal responsibility be held against the publisher, or author, for any damages, reparation, or monetary loss due to the information contained within this book. Either directly or indirectly.

Legal Notice:

This book is copyright protected. This book is only for personal use. You cannot amend, distribute, sell, use, quote or paraphrase any part, or the content within this book, without the consent of the author or publisher.

Disclaimer Notice:

Please note the information contained within this document is for educational and entertainment purposes only. All effort has been executed to present accurate, up to date, and reliable, complete information. No warranties of any kind are declared or implied. Readers acknowledge that the author is not engaging in the rendering of legal, financial, medical or professional advice. The content within this book has been derived from various sources. Please consult a licensed professional before attempting any techniques outlined in this book.

By reading this document, the reader agrees that under no circumstances is the author responsible for any losses, direct or indirect, which are incurred as a result of the use of information contained within this document, including, but not limited to, — errors, omissions, or inaccuracies.

Table of Contents:

INTRODUCTION

PALEOLITHIC DIET

Let's talk about the return to the origins of man, what was once the food to eat, unprocessed and especially not CULTIVATED!

PROTEINS AND FATS

The Paleolithic diet had a higher protein component than that recommended today and differed significantly from the latter. Meat was lean game, poorer and very different in the composition of fats than today's meat. Moreover, this food was rich in Omega-3 fats, today almost absent in the meat of animals raised on feed (a clear difference from those raised free). Fats are however an essential and important component of the paleolithic diet.

CARBOHYDRATES

As far as the use of carbohydrates is concerned, as a source of energy and to restore the acid-base balance of the body, Paleolithic man ate fruit and vegetables, which lead (compared to pasta, rice and bread) to a lower release of insulin, consequently to a lower synthesis of fats. Carbohydrates with a high glycemic index, in fact, those derived from cereals, are responsible for the rapid rise in the concentration of glucose in the blood (blood sugar), an event that triggers the "perverse mechanism of insulin".

WHAT TO EAT

So, to recap, the tips for a good paleolithic diet are:

1) **Have many small meals and not a few large ones**: this also reduces hormonal (insulin) stimulation compared to that caused by larger, more concentrated meals.
2) **Eat red or white meat**: even if today's meat is treated compared to millions of years ago and loses many nutritional values compared to the paleolithic one; it is not a coincidence that farm animals are given feed with cereals in it, when they were free, however, they ate what nature had imposed.
3) **Eat carbohydrates** taken from fruits and vegetables, avoiding pasta, bread, cookies, rusks, rice and all derivatives of cereals.

4) **Dissociate foods correctly**, i.e. avoid mixing different proteins, in this way each food will be better digested and absorbed by the body.
5) **Do physical activity**: Paleolithic man went hunting to get food, he didn't sit on a sofa watching TV, and made a fight to kill the animal; now instead we go to the supermarket and everything is already ready, so it is very important to do some sport.

With this diet I was able to "bring back to the roots" many people in a short time, devastated by dietary regimens that unfortunately today's society imposes on us.

Happy re-entry into today's civilization or
happy beginning of a New Era...
THE PALEO!

WHY THE BOOK SPECIFICALLY FOR WOMEN

How easy it is to fall into banality when talking about women in the kitchen. The chauvinist phrase is just around the corner, perhaps hidden in the folds of a fake smile.

How many times have we heard that the restaurant kitchen is too hard for us women, so petite and weak?
How many times have we heard the opposite, that women are better because they have hospitality in their blood, sensitivity and love for others?

What makes a great chef is sensitivity, regardless of gender, but even today restaurant kitchens are an extremely macho world, a world locked in a bubble of camaraderie that is harmful to all. Think about this fact: still today only 4% of Michelin Stars in the world are women, a derisory figure, almost offensive. Women with 3 Stars are very few, even though fortunately in the last five years things have slightly improved.

Yet there are women all over the world who have made and are making restaurant history, with exceptional results that should have convinced the world's critics a long time ago to focus on the "asexuality" of cooking, that is, to think only of the dish and not of those who prepare it. A few years ago at the presentation of the "Rossa" in Italy, the only woman awarded was Karime Lopez, the first Mexican cook to have this honor. When they asked her why she was the only female, her answer was courageous: "There are women in the kitchen, they are good, it is you who have to look for them better".

We are perfectly capable of cooking great recipes, for me it is a pleasure to be in the kitchen, my life is the kitchen!

What I want to tell you is: take a cue from these recipes and take the time to let your crativity explode. I have given you a list of recipes, you can modify them to your liking and make tasty masterpieces!

Good luck!
Tess

Important:
To lose weight, however, you need to combine your diet with exercise, such as walking, going to the gym, biking and more. This cookbook lists a number of Paleo recipes that are not intended to replace the advice of a nutritionist.

Everything that truly makes us happy is quite simple – love, sex and food!

- Meryl Streep -

MEASUREMENT CONVERSION

Volume Equivalents (Liquid)

Type	US Standard (ounces)	Metric
2 tablespoons	1 fl. oz.	30 mL
¼ cup	2 fl. oz.	60 mL
½ cup	4 fl. oz.	120 mL
1 cup	8 fl. oz.	240mL

Volume Equivalents (Dry)

Type	Metric
¼ teaspoon	1 mL
½ teaspoon	2 mL
1 teaspoon	5 mL
1 tablespoon	15 mL
¼ cup	59 mL
½ cup	118 mL
1 cup	235 mL

Oven Temperatures

Fahrenheit (°F)	Celsius (°C)
250	120
300	150
325	165
350	180
375	190
400	200
425	220
450	230

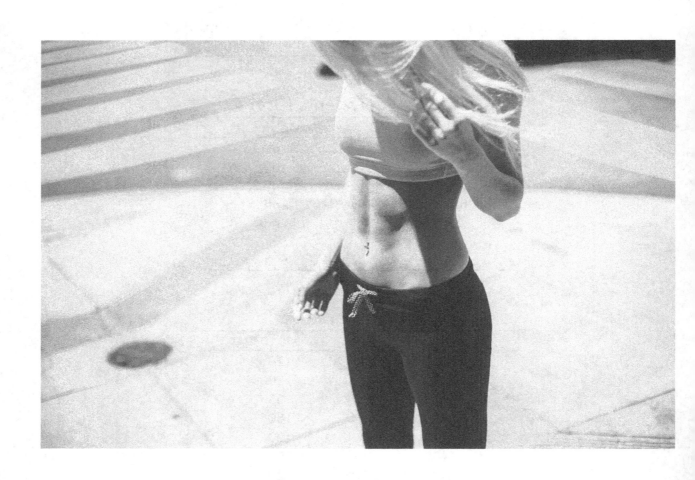

THE 10 GOLDEN RULES

1. Keep 10 Paleo foods on hand at all times, in your office, in your home, in your car, in your wallet. Nuts and pumpkin seeds are great options.
2. Plan a menu of meals for the week. This will help you know what to buy at the grocery store and ensure you have a delicious, healthy meal every day.
3. Cook large portions. This will help you have ready, healthy food on hand for a couple of days.
4. Don't keep foods in the house that are not paleo friendly. If this will be on hand, it will be a great temptation.
5. If you find it hard to eliminate some foods that you have a sweet tooth for that aren't 100% paleo, start decreasing the portions.
6. Don't run out of food. Can't cook anything? Don't have anything paleo at home to eat that's healthy? Are you hungry? Don't let this happen to you, it's very easy in these cases to give in to temptation.
7. Try new ingredients and seasonings. Seasonings are great for improving the taste of a dish and trying new innovative dishes.
8. If possible, freeze some of the foods you've cooked. This way, you have something on hand in the freezer, so if you don't have time to go grocery shopping, you won't starve.
9. Fall in love with plants, which are essential to your health and fitness. Don't be afraid to try new vegetables in different colors.
10. Avoid cooking the same things over and over again, you'll end up bored with your diet.

Enjoy the paleo diet and all your meals!

8

PALEO RECIPES FOR WOMEN

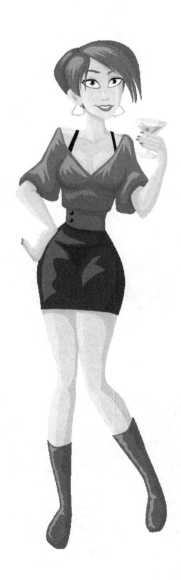

CRAWFISH IN RED SAUCE

Serv.: 10| **Prep.:** 25m | **Cook:** 50m

Ingredients:
- ✓ 3 tablespoons vegetable oil
- ✓ 1 tablespoon minced garlic
- ✓ 1 large onion, chopped
- ✓ 1/4 cup chopped green bell pepper
- ✓ 1/4 cup chopped celery
- ✓ 1 (8 ounce) can tomato sauce
- ✓ 1 (14.5 ounce) can whole peeled tomatoes, undrained and chopped
- ✓ 1/2 (14.5 ounce) can diced tomatoes with green chile peppers (such as RO*TEL®)
- ✓ Salt and pepper to taste
- ✓ 5 pounds cooked and peeled whole crawfish tails

Directions: Put vegetable oil in a large saucepan and heat it over medium heat. Mix in bell pepper, garlic, celery, and onion and cook for 10 minutes until the celery is tender and the onion is translucent. Stir in chopped tomatoes together with their juice, diced tomatoes, and tomato sauce. Season the mixture with salt and pepper to taste. Boil the mixture over medium-high heat. Decrease the heat and let it simmer for 30 minutes. Mix in crawfish tails. Simmer for 5-10 minutes until hot.

FRUIT SMOOTHIE

Serv.: 1| **Prep.:** 10m | **Cook:** 0

Ingredients:
- ✓ 1 1/2 cups crushed ice
- ✓ 1 banana, chopped
- ✓ 1 kiwi, peeled and chopped
- ✓ 1/2 cup chopped strawberries
- ✓ 1/2 cup chopped pineapple
- ✓ 1/4 cup cream of coconut
- ✓ 1 tablespoon coconut flakes for garnish

Directions: Using a blender, mix kiwi, pineapple, strawberries and banana together with ice and cream of coconut. Blend and mix until it becomes smooth. Transfer it into the glass and decorate it with coconut flakes before serving.

CREOLE PORK SHANKS WITH SWEET POTATO GRAVY

Serv.: 4| **Prep.:** 25m | **Cook:** 6h

Ingredients:
- ✓ 2 sweet potatoes
- ✓ 1 teaspoon vegetable oil
- ✓ 4 pork shanks, cut in half
- ✓ 1/2 teaspoon ground black pepper
- ✓ 1/4 teaspoon cayenne pepper
- ✓ 1/4 cup olive oil
- ✓ 1 medium onion, chopped
- ✓ 3 celery ribs, chopped
- ✓ 1 small green bell pepper, chopped
- ✓ 4 garlic cloves, minced
- ✓ 4 cups Swanson® Chicken Broth, plus more if needed
- ✓ 2 (14.5 ounce) cans diced tomatoes
- ✓ 3 bay leaves
- ✓ 1 teaspoon dried thyme
- ✓ 1/4 teaspoon cayenne pepper
- ✓ 1/2 teaspoon black pepper

Directions: Preheat an oven to 175°C/350°F; rub vegetable oil on sweet potatoes. In aluminum foil, wrap.
In preheated oven, put sweet potatoes; bake for 1 hour till soft. Peel then cut into 1-in. chunks when cool enough to handle.
Season all sides of pork shanks with cayenne pepper and black pepper.
Heat olive oil in big skillet on medium-high heat; cook all sides of shanks for 10 minutes in total till all sides are nicely browned. Put pork shanks into slow cooker.
Sauté garlic, bell pepper, celery and onion in skillet, scraping browned bits from the bottom; cook on medium heat for 5 minutes till soft.
Mix diced tomatoes and 4 cups of Swanson® Chicken Broth in; boil. Add thyme and bay leaves; simmer for 10 minutes till mixture slightly reduces. Put mixture into slow cooker with pork shanks;

cook for 6 hours on high till tender. Put pork shanks onto a platter; to keep warm, tent with foil.
Take 1/2 veggies out of the cooking liquid; discard/keep for another use. Put all liquid and leftover veggies into a food processor/blender; put cooked sweet potato chunks in; process for 1 minute till smooth.
Add 2 tbsp. chicken broth at a time till you get your desired gravy consistency in case the gravy is too thick.
Put sweet potato gravy on top of pork shank servings.

CREOLO COCKTAIL

Serv.: 1| **Prep.:** 5m | **Cook:** 0

Ingredients:
- ✓ 1 lemon, cut into 4 wedges
- ✓ 5 leaves fresh mint
- ✓ 1/4 fluid ounce agave nectar
- ✓ 1 cup crushed ice
- ✓ 1 1/2 fluid ounces spiced rum
- ✓ 1 fluid ounce club soda, or as needed
- ✓ 1 sprig fresh mint

Directions: In a lowball glass, muddle together agave nectar, mint leaves and 3 lemon wedges until aromatic. Put in rum and crushed ice, then put club soda on top. Pour the mixture back froth into a cocktail shaker or mixing glass until mixed.
Serve in a lowball glass decorated with a lemon wedge and a sprig of fresh mint.

PORK SAUSAGE PATTIES WITH APRICOTS AND PISTACHIOS

Serv.: 4| **Prep.:** 20m | **Cook:** 12m

Ingredients:
- ✓ 1 1/2 pounds coarsely ground pork
- ✓ 2 teaspoons kosher salt
- ✓ 1 teaspoon black pepper
- ✓ 1 pinch cayenne pepper
- ✓ 1 pinch dried sage
- ✓ 1 teaspoon very finely sliced fresh sage leaves
- ✓ 1/4 cup chopped pistachio nuts
- ✓ 2 tablespoons diced dried apricots
- ✓ 1/2 pound caul fat

Directions: In the mixing bowl, whisk together apricots, pistachios, fresh sage, dried sage, cayenne pepper, pepper, salt, and sausage using a fork till just combined. Split into 4 parts and form into patties that are roughly three quarters in. in thickness.
Chop the caul fat into pieces that are roughly 2-3 in. bigger than the crepinette patty. Wrap the patty in caul fat with the ends tucked on the bottom. The patties should be covered entirely. If the caul fat pieces are small, overlap them to cover each patty entirely. Trim off any redundant caul fat, as you want. Add the patties onto the dish and use the plastic wrap to cover up; keep in the refrigerator overnight.
Heat 1 tbsp. of oil on medium heat in the skillet. Add the crepinettes smooth side facing downward into the pan. Allow to brown for 3 - 4 minutes per side. Blot some of rendered fat using the wadded up paper towel. Add in a splash of the white wine; cover up. Cook while covered till the inside of patties reaches 63 degrees C/145 degrees F in temperature, or 5 more minutes. Remove the cover and turn the crepinettes to coat along with pan brownings and to decrease some of the wine.

CRISPY PORK CARNITAS

Serv.: 6| **Prep.:** 15m | **Cook:** 3h40m

Ingredients:
- ✓ 3 pounds boneless pork butt (shoulder)
- ✓ 8 cloves garlic, peeled
- ✓ 1/4 cup olive oil
- ✓ 1 orange, juiced, orange parts of peel removed and sliced into thin strips
- ✓ 1 tablespoon kosher salt
- ✓ 2 bay leaves, torn in half
- ✓ 1 teaspoon ground black pepper
- ✓ 1 teaspoon ground cumin
- ✓ 3/4 teaspoon ground cinnamon
- ✓ 1/2 teaspoon Chinese 5-spice powder

Directions: Set oven to 135°C (or 275°F) and start preheating.

Skim fat off the pork; cube pork meat into 2" pieces and coarsely chop fat.

In a bowl, combine 5-spice powder, cinnamon, cumin, black pepper, bay leaves, salt, orange juice, orange peel, olive oil, garlic with pork until pork is thoroughly coated. Bring mixture to a 9x13" baking dish. Set the dish on a baking sheet and tightly wrap heavy-duty aluminum foil around.

Bake pork for 3 1/2 hours in prepared oven until pork is easily flaked with a fork.

Place oven rack in a 6"-distance away from the heat; start preheating the oven's broiler.

Set meat onto a colander placed over a bowl. Take out orange peels, bay leaves and garlic from baking dish and stream accumulated juices from the baking dish onto the meat placed in colander into the bowl. Take meat back to the baking dish and pour accumulated juices onto each piece of meat. Cook meat for 3 minutes in the prepared broiler. Pour more accumulated juices onto the meat and keep broiling for another 3-5 minutes until crisped. Bring pork to serving dish and top with more accumulated juices.

CRISPY AND TENDER BAKED CHICKEN THIGHS

Serv.: 8| **Prep.:** 10m | **Cook:** 1h

Ingredients:
Cooking spray:
- ✓ 8 bone-in chicken thighs with skin
- ✓ 1/4 teaspoon garlic salt
- ✓ 1/4 teaspoon onion salt
- ✓ 1/4 teaspoon dried oregano
- ✓ 1/4 teaspoon ground thyme
- ✓ 1/4 teaspoon paprika
- ✓ 1/4 teaspoon ground black pepper

Directions: Set oven to 350°F (175°C) to preheat.

Line aluminum foil over a baking sheet and apply cooking spray all over.

Place chicken thighs on the prepared baking sheet.

In a small container with a lid, mix together pepper, paprika, thyme, oregano, onion salt, and garlic salt. Cover the container with a lid and shake until spices are well blended. Scatter spice mixture generously over chicken thighs.

Bake chicken for about 60 minutes in the preheated oven until no pink remain at the bones, chicken juices run clear, and skin is crispy. An instant-read thermometer pinned near the bone should register 165°F (74°C).

CRISPY, SPICY CAULIFLOWER PANCAKES

Serv.: 12| **Prep.:** 15m | **Cook:** 36m

Ingredients:
- ✓ 1 tablespoon coconut oil
- ✓ 1 teaspoon olive oil
- ✓ 2 cups grated cauliflower
- ✓ 2 tablespoons finely chopped onion
- ✓ 1 clove garlic, minced
- ✓ 1 cup 1% cottage cheese, drained
- ✓ 1/4 cup egg whites
- ✓ 1 tablespoon hot pepper sauce (such as Frank's RedHot®), or to taste
- ✓ 2 teaspoons dried parsley
- ✓ 1 teaspoon dried oregano
- ✓ 1/4 teaspoon garlic powder

Directions: Prepare the oven by preheating to 350°F (175°C). Use coconut oil to grease a 12-cup muffin tin.

Put the olive oil in a skillet over medium heat. Put in the garlic, onion, and cauliflower. Stir and cook for 6-8 minutes until the cauliflower turns slightly translucent and garlic and onions are tender. Transfer to a bowl allows it to cool.

In a blender, combine garlic powder, oregano, parsley, hot sauce, egg whites, and cottage cheese; blend until smooth. Place into the bowl of cauliflower mixture; blend fully. Scoop mixture equally into the greased muffin cups and push down so pancakes are flat and equal.

Place in the preheated oven and bake for approximately 30 minutes until tops and edges are crispy and golden.

CUBAN GOULASH

Serv.: 6| Prep.: 20m | Cook: 40m

Ingredients:
- ✓ 1 tablespoon vegetable oil
- ✓ 1 pound boneless pork roast, cubed
- ✓ 1 pound onions, diced
- ✓ 1 pound bananas, peeled and diced
- ✓ 1 (16 ounce) can diced tomatoes with juice
- ✓ Cayenne pepper to taste
- ✓ Salt and ground black pepper to taste

Directions: Over medium heat, heat oil in a large skillet, add pork and then brown on all sides. Stir in onions and then cook while stirring until tender. Combine the tomatoes with juice and bananas into the skillet. Heat to boil, decrease the heat to medium low and let simmer for 30 minutes while stirring often until the pork becomes very tender. Season with pepper, salt and cayenne pepper.

CURRIED BEEF

Serv.: 4| Prep.: 10m | Cook: 35m

Ingredients:
- ✓ 2 tablespoons vegetable oil
- ✓ 1 pound stew beef, cubed
- ✓ 1 1/2 teaspoons curry powder
- ✓ 1/2 teaspoon salt
- ✓ 1/2 teaspoon ground black pepper
- ✓ 2 tablespoons tomato paste
- ✓ 1/4 cup water
- ✓ 1 onion, chopped
- ✓ 2 stalks celery, chopped
- ✓ 1/2 cup raisins
- ✓ 1 apple - peeled, cored, and chopped

Directions: Heat the oil in a large skillet over medium heat. Place the meat in the hot oil and sauté until well browned on all sides. Sprinkle the curry powder, salt, and ground black pepper over the meat and stir well.
Beat water and tomato paste together in a small bowl, then mix the mixture into the skillet. Stir in raisins, celery, and onion, turn down the heat to low and simmer until the beef becomes tender, half an hour.
Mix the apple into the skillet and simmer until the sauce becomes thick and the apple becomes tender, 5 minutes longer.

CURRY SALMON WITH MANGO

Serv.: 4| Prep.: 15m | Cook: 15m

Ingredients:
- ✓ 1 (1 pound) fillet salmon fillet
- ✓ 1/4 cup avocado oil
- ✓ 1 teaspoon curry powder
- ✓ Salt to taste
- ✓ 1 mango - peeled, seeded, and diced
- ✓ 1/4 cup diced red onion
- ✓ 1 small serrano pepper, diced
- ✓ 1 small bunch cilantro leaves
- ✓ 1 lime

Directions: Set oven to 400°F or 200°C. Use aluminum foil to line cookie sheet.
Put the salmon in cookie sheet and cover salmon with the foil. Crumple the edges to seal.
Bake for about 15 minutes until fish flakes easily using fork.
Meanwhile, combine curry powder, avocado oil and salt in a small bowl. Pour dressing over the salmon and top with red onion, serrano pepper and diced mango. Before serving, squeeze lime and sprinkle cilantro on top.

CZECH CABBAGE DISH

Serv.: 10| Prep.: 20m | Cook: 10m

Ingredients:
- ✓ 1 large head cabbage, shredded
- ✓ 1/4 pound bacon, chopped
- ✓ 1 tablespoon vegetable oil
- ✓ 1 small onion, chopped
- ✓ 1 stalk celery, chopped
- ✓ 1/4 cup chopped green bell pepper
- ✓ 3 tablespoons white vinegar
- ✓ 1/2 teaspoon salt

1 teaspoon black pepper

Directions: Boil a large pot filled with lightly salted water and then blanche the cabbage into the water briefly. Remove them from water and drain them right away.

Cook the bacon in a large skillet over medium heat until brown and opaque. Remove from the heat and let it drain on paper towels.

Discard all the bacon grease except for 1 tbsp. of it. Add 1 tbsp. of vegetable oil to the skillet. Heat the oil over medium heat. Add the bell pepper, celery, and onion. Cook until crisp-tender.

Mix the bacon, salt, pepper, prepared cabbage, vinegar, and sautéed vegetable mix with oil in a large bowl. Toss the mixture well and serve while warm. You can also chill the mixture and serve it later.

SHREDDED BEEF

Serv.: 4| **Prep.:** 10m | **Cook:** 5h

Ingredients:
- 1 1/2 pounds rump roast
- 1 1/4 cups water
- Garlic powder, or to taste
- Salt and ground black pepper to taste

Directions: Generously season rump roast with pepper, salt and garlic powder; place into the crock of a slow cooker. Pour the water into the crock. Cook for 5 hours on high. Take the roast away onto a cutting board; use 2 forks to shred.

BEST HAROSET

Serv.: 4| **Prep.:** 10m | **Cook:** 0

Ingredients:
- 3 apples - peeled, cored, and diced
- 1 cup walnuts, chopped
- 1 cup pecans, chopped
- 1 cup kosher red wine
- 1 teaspoon cinnamon

Directions: In a big bowl, mix wine, pecans,

walnuts and apples together. Use cinnamon to season. Stir the mixture and put it in the refrigerator for about 30 minutes until chilled.

ROAST PORK PUERTO RICAN STYLE

Serv.: 8| **Prep.:** 15m | **Cook:** 4h

Ingredients:
- 1/4 cup olive oil
- 3 tablespoons white vinegar
- 10 cloves garlic, or more to taste
- 2 tablespoons dried oregano
- 1 tablespoon salt
- 1 1/2 teaspoons ground black pepper
- 5 pounds pork shoulder, trimmed of excess fat

Directions: In a mortar and pestle, mix black pepper, salt, oregano, garlic, vinegar and olive oil together before mashing them up to a paste. Use a little knife to cut some slits deep into the pork then insert the paste into slits. Place any leftover paste atop pork, rubbing it in. Put the pork into a plastic roasting bag then set it on a rack inside of a roasting pan. Leave it marinating for a minimum of 8 hours up to 48 hours.

After getting the pork out from the fridge, remove the cover and let it cool down for an hour or two hours until it's at room temperature.

Preheat the oven to 300°F (150°C).

Put the meat into the preheated oven, roasting for around 2 hours with the skin side facing down until it becomes a nice golden brown. Turn the pork around. Proceed to roast with the skin side up for about 2-4 hours until the juices start running clear. It's done when the instant-read thermometer reads a minimum of 145°F (63°C) when put into the middle of the pork. If desired, serve with sweet plantains, salad or beans and rice.

DARK CHOCOLATE ALMOND ROCKS

Serv.: 20| **Prep.:** 10m | **Cook:** 8m

Ingredients:
- 1/2 cup almonds, crushed into chunks

✓ 7 ounces dark chocolate chips (50% cacao)

Directions: In big skillet, spread almonds; toast for 3-5 minutes till starting to brown on medium heat. Put almonds in bowl.
In top of double boiler above simmering water, melt chocolate, frequently mixing and scraping side down to avoid scorching for 5 minutes; take off heat. Put almonds in; mix till coated evenly.
On waxed paper-lined plate, drop spoonfuls of chocolate-almond mixture.
Chill for 10 minutes till set.

DARK CHOCOLATE ESPRESSO PALEO MUG CAKE

Serv.: 1 | **Prep.:** 5m | **Cook:** 2m

Ingredients:
✓ 4 ounces dark chocolate chips
✓ 1 tablespoon coconut oil
✓ 2 tablespoons water
✓ 1 tablespoon blanched almond flour
✓ 1 tablespoon coconut flour
✓ 1 pinch baking soda
✓ 1 egg
✓ 1 tablespoon brewed espresso

Directions: In a microwave-safe mug, mix the coconut oil and chocolate chips. Let it heat in the microwave for about 30 seconds, until it melts. Whisk the baking soda, coconut flour, almond flour and water into the chocolate mixture, until well blended. Add brewed espresso and egg, then whisk until it becomes smooth.
Let it heat it in the microwave for about 90 seconds, until the cake is cooked through. Allow it to cool for about 2 minutes prior to serving.

DASHI STOCK

Serv.: 8 | **Prep.:** 5m | **Cook:** 5m

Ingredients:
✓ 1 ounce dashi Kombu
✓ 1 quart water
✓ 1/2 cup bonito flakes

Directions: Use a paper towel to clean any dirt from the kombu, but be careful not to scuff the white powdery deposits on seaweed. In a saucepan, put water and the kombu, allow to soak for about 30 minutes to get softened.
Next, remove the seaweed from the water, trim some lengthways splits into the leaf. Put them back into the water and boil. When the water begins to boil, take the seaweed out to prevent the stock from getting bitter.
Stir the bonito flakes into the kombu-flavored broth, boil again, then remove the pan from the heat. Let the water cool down. Once the bonito flakes have sunk to the bottom, use a coffee filter or a strainer lined with cheesecloth to strain the dashi.

ROAST PORK FOR TACOS

Serv.: 12 | **Prep.:** 15m | **Cook:** 4h

Ingredients:
✓ 4 pounds pork shoulder roast
✓ 2 (4 ounce) cans diced green chilies, drained
✓ 1/4 cup chili powder
✓ 1 teaspoon dried oregano
✓ 1 teaspoon taco seasoning
✓ 2 teaspoons minced garlic
✓ 1 1/2 teaspoons salt, or to taste

Directions: Set the oven to 300 degrees F (150 degrees C) to preheat.
Place roast atop a big piece of aluminum foil. Stir together garlic, taco seasoning, oregano, chili powder, and green chiles together in a small bowl; rub the mixture on the roast. Wrap the roast in the foil to completely cover it, using more foil if needed. Put it on a roasting rack set in a baking dish. Otherwise, you can just place a cookie sheet on an oven rack below to catch leaks.
Roast in prepared oven until the meat falls apart, around 3 1/2-4 hours. Cook the roast until it reaches a minimum of 145 degrees F or 63 degrees C. Take out of the oven and use 2 forks to shred the roast into small pieces, season to taste with salt.

DEEP FRIED SALT AND PEPPER SHRIMP

Serv.: 8 | **Prep.:** 15m | **Cook:** 15m

Ingredients:
- ✓ 1 pound large shrimp in shells, peeled and deveined
- ✓ 3/4 teaspoon sea salt (such as Diamond Crystal®)
- ✓ 1/2 teaspoon freshly ground black pepper
- ✓ 1/2 teaspoon Chinese 5-spice powder
- ✓ 4 cups vegetable oil for frying

Directions: Cut off the hard pointed area right above the tail and the feathery legs of each shrimp. Rinse the shrimp; dry thoroughly.
In a small bowl, mix together 5-spice powder, pepper and salt.
In a heavy pot or a wok over high heat, heat oil till your deep fry thermometer attains 400°F (200°C). Cook the shrimp in the hot oil, around 5 per batch, for around 1 minute, or till the shrimp are cooked through and bright pink. Using a slotted spoon, take the shrimp away; remove onto a plate lined with paper towels. Turn the oil temperature back to 400°F (200°C) before each new batch.
Pour off the oil in the wok; place the wok over medium-high heat; put in the spice mix and the deep-fried shrimp; cook while stirring constantly for 30 seconds to 1 minute, or till fragrant.

DEEP FRIED TURKEY

Serv.: 16 | **Prep.:** 30m | **Cook:** 45m

Ingredients:
- ✓ 3 gallons peanut oil for frying, or as needed
- ✓ 1 (12 pound) whole turkey, neck and giblets removed
- ✓ 1/4 cup Creole seasoning
- ✓ 1 white onion

Directions: Preheat oil to 400 degrees F (200 degrees C) in a big turkey fryer or a stockpot. Make sure not to fill the pot with too much oil or it will spill. Prepare a big platter and line it with paper towels or food-safe paper bags. Pat the rinsed turkey with paper towels until thoroughly dry. Massage the outside and cavity of the bird with Creole seasoning. See to it that the neck hole has a two-inch opening to ensure that the oil will reach the inside of the turkey. Put the turkey and whole onions in the drain basket, positioning the turkey neck end first. Carefully submerge the basket into the hot oil, completely submerging the turkey. Fry the turkey for 45 minutes or 3 1/2 minutes per pound, make sure that the oil stays at 350 degrees F (175 degrees C) throughout the cooking process. Slowly and carefully lift the basket from oil and drain the turkey. Thermometer inserted inside thickest area of thigh should read 180 degrees F (80 degrees C). Drain excess oil on prepared platter.

DEEP FRIED TURKEY BREAST

Serv.: 12 | **Prep.:** 5m | **Cook:** 25m

Ingredients:
- ✓ 2 tablespoons sea salt
- ✓ 1 tablespoon red pepper flakes
- ✓ 1 tablespoon freshly ground black pepper
- ✓ 1 tablespoon granulated garlic
- ✓ 1 tablespoon chili powder
- ✓ 1 (7 pound) turkey breast
- ✓ 2 gallons canola oil for frying

Directions: In a plastic container with a matching lid, combine the red pepper flakes, chili powder, granulated garlic, sea salt, and black pepper. Seal the container with its lid and shake until the seasonings are well-combined.
Rub the spice mixture all over the turkey breast until well-coated. Use an aluminum foil to wrap the breast; refrigerate for 24 hours.
Get the breast from the refrigerator and allow it to stand at room temperature.
Meanwhile, heat the oil in a pot with a lid (enough to hold the oil and breast to 325°F or 165°C).
Add the breast into the hot oil. Cover the pot with its lid. Fry the turkey for 25 minutes until its juices run clear and the turkey is no longer pinkish in the center. Make sure that the inserted instant-read thermometer into the turkey's center should read at least 165°F (74°C).

DELICIOUS SWEET POTATO FRIES

Serv.: 2 | **Prep.:** 10m | **Cook:** 20m

Ingredients:
- ✓ 2 sweet potatoes, peeled and cut into 1/2-inch slices
- ✓ 1 tablespoon coconut oil, melted
- ✓ 1 teaspoon ground cumin
- ✓ 1/2 teaspoon garlic powder
- ✓ Salt and ground black pepper to taste
- ✓ 1/2 teaspoon paprika
- ✓ 2 tablespoons chopped fresh cilantro (optional)

Directions: Preheat the oven to 230°C or 450°F.
Onto a baking sheet, lay sweet potatoes. Sprinkle coconut oil on top of sweet potatoes; season with pepper, salt, garlic powder and cumin.
In the prepped oven, bake for 20 to 25 minutes till soft in the middle, flipping from time to time. Jazz up with cilantro and paprika.

DELICIOUS AND EASY PRIME RIB

Serv.: 14 | **Prep.:** 15m | **Cook:** 3h30m

Ingredients:
- ✓ 1 (7 pound) bone-in prime rib, trimmed and retied to the bone
- ✓ 8 cloves garlic
- ✓ 2 tablespoons olive oil
- ✓ 2 teaspoons kosher salt
- ✓ 2 teaspoons freshly ground black pepper
- ✓ 1 ounce fresh rosemary, or to taste
- ✓ 1 ounce fresh thyme, or to taste

Directions: Start preheating the oven at 350°F (175°C).
Cut several slits into the top of prime rib; press garlic cloves into slits. Brush olive oil over the prime rib and flavor with pepper and salt. Place thyme sprigs and rosemary sprigs atop prime rib and put into a roasting pan.
Bake in the prepared oven for 3 1/2 to 4 hours until the outside is browned and the center is pink. An instant-read thermometer should show at least 125°F (52°C) when inserted into the center. Let the prime rib rest for 15 minutes before cutting.

FISH BAKED IN A SALT CRUST

Serv.: 4 | **Prep.:** 30m | **Cook:** 30m

Ingredients:
- ✓ 2 pounds salt
- ✓ 7 bay leaves
- ✓ 2 pounds whole rainbow trout, gutted and cleaned, heads and tails still on
- ✓ 2 sprigs fresh cilantro, or more to taste
- ✓ 2 sprigs fresh parsley, or more to taste
- ✓ 2 sprigs fresh dill, or more to taste

Directions: Preheat the oven to 200 degrees C/400 degrees F. Line aluminum foil on a baking sheet.
Spread 1/4 - 1/2-lb. salt on aluminum foil to around the same shape as the fish. Put bay leaves on salt. Put fish on top. Stuff dill, parsley and cilantro into fish cavity. Firmly pack down leftover salt on fish. Leave tail and head exposed.
Bake in preheated oven for 30 minutes until salt crust becomes golden.
Remove fish from oven. Crack open salt crust carefully. Remove the top. Peel off fish skin to expose flesh. Use a spatula/fish knife to lift top fillet off the bones. In one piece, remove bones by lifting from the tail then pull upwards towards the head. Lift bottom fillet out with a spatula/knife.

TILAPIA FILIPINO SOUR BROTH DISH

Serv.: 4 | **Prep.:** 5m | **Cook:** 10m

Ingredients:
- ✓ 1/2 pound tilapia fillets, cut into chunks
- ✓ 1 small head bok choy, chopped
- ✓ 2 medium tomatoes, cut into chunks
- ✓ 1 cup thinly sliced daikon radish
- ✓ 1/4 cup tamarind paste
- ✓ 3 cups water
- ✓ 2 dried red chile peppers (optional)

Directions: Mix radish, tomatoes, bok choy, and tilapia in a medium pot. Mix water and tamarind paste; add into the pot. Mix in the chili peppers if you want. Make it boil then cook for 5 minutes, or just until the fish is cooked well. Even fish that is frozen will be cooked in less than ten minutes. Keep from overcooking or else the fish will fall apart. Scoop into bowls to serve.

FLAT IRON STEAK

Serv.: 2| **Prep.:** 5m | **Cook:** 6m

Ingredients:
- ✓ 2 (8 ounce) flat iron steaks
- ✓ 1/2 teaspoon lemon pepper seasoning, or to taste
- ✓ 1/2 teaspoon onion powder, or to taste
- ✓ 1/2 teaspoon garlic powder, or to taste

Directions: Sprinkle garlic powder, onion powder and lemon pepper on both sides of the steak to season. Use plastic wrap to wrap and marinate in the refrigerator for at least 2 hours.
Set the grill to medium-high heat to preheat and let the steaks to come to room temperature. Remove wrap and put on the prepared grill. Cook to the degree of doneness you prefer, about 3 minutes on each side for medium rare. Before serving, let steaks sit for a few minutes.

FLAT IRON STEAK WITH MUSHROOMS

Serv.: 3| **Prep.:** 15m | **Cook:** 15m

Ingredients:
- ✓ 3 tablespoons vegetable oil
- ✓ Salt and pepper to taste
- ✓ 3 (6 ounce) flat iron steaks
- ✓ 3 shallots, thinly sliced
- ✓ 6 cloves garlic, peeled
- ✓ 4 cups sliced white mushrooms
- ✓ 1/4 cup balsamic vinegar
- ✓ 3/4 cup full-bodied red wine

Directions: Set the oven at 350°F (175°C) and start preheating.
In a large skillet over medium heat, heat oil. Slice flat iron steak into individual portions if necessary. Season both sides with pepper and salt. Fry the

steaks for 2-3 minutes on each side, till well-browned on both sides. Take away from the skillet; place on an oven-proof dish. Put the steaks into the oven; continue cooking.
Put whole cloves of garlic and shallots into the hot skillet. Cook while stirring over medium heat till the shallots begin to brown. Put in mushrooms; cook while stirring for 5-10 minutes, or till they shrink some.
Pour in balsamic vinegar; stir to discard any browned bits on the bottom of the skillet. Transfer in red wine; simmer over medium heat for a few minutes.
Transfer the steaks back to the skillet; cook for around 5 minutes if at all, or till the internal temperature registers 135-140°F (60°C). Take the whole pan away from the heat; allow to sit to reach your desired doneness, or till the steaks attain an internal temperature of 145°F (63°C).

FLOURLESS CREPE TORTILLAS

Serv.: 9| **Prep.:** 10m | **Cook:** 1m

Ingredients:
- ✓ 2 tablespoons water
- ✓ 2 teaspoons ghee (clarified butter), melted
- ✓ 4 eggs
- ✓ 1/2 cup tapioca flour
- ✓ 2 teaspoons coconut flour
- ✓ 1 pinch sea salt

Directions: Combine ghee and water together in a bowl. Whisk in egg until frothy. Add coconut flour, sea salt, and tapioca flour and mix until smooth. Place an 8-inches nonstick skillet over medium-low heat. Drop 2 tbsp. of the batter into the hot skillet and slowly swirl the skillet to coat the bottom evenly. Let it cook for 30 seconds. Flip it over and cook the other side for another 30 seconds. Place it into a plate. Do the same with the remaining batter.

FLOURLESS DOUBLE CHOCOLATE CHIP ZUCCHINI MUFFINS

Serv.: 8| **Prep.:** 30m | **Cook:** 25m

Ingredients:
- ✓ 1/2 cup almond butter
- ✓ 1 ripe banana, mashed
- ✓ 1/4 cup unsweetened cocoa powder
- ✓ 2 tablespoons ground flax seeds
- ✓ 1 tablespoon honey
- ✓ 1 teaspoon vanilla extract
- ✓ 1/2 teaspoon baking soda
- ✓ 1 cup finely grated zucchini, excess moisture squeezed out
- ✓ 1/4 cup semisweet chocolate chips
- ✓ 1/4 cup bittersweet chocolate chips, or to taste

Directions: Set the oven to 375°F or 190°C for preheating. Use an aluminum foil liners to line the muffin cups.

In a bowl, combine the banana, ground flax seeds, vanilla extract, baking soda, honey, cocoa powder, and almond butter until the batter is well-blended. Fold in semisweet chocolate chips and zucchini. Spoon the batter into the prepared muffin cups. Top each cups with bittersweet chocolate chips. Allow them to bake inside the preheated oven for 25 minutes until an inserted toothpick on its center comes out clean. Transfer muffins on a wire rack to cool completely.

FOOLPROOF RIB ROAST

Serv.: 6| **Prep.:** 5m | **Cook:** 5h

Ingredients:
- ✓ 1 (5 pound) standing beef rib roast
- ✓ 2 teaspoons salt
- ✓ 1 teaspoon ground black pepper
- ✓ 1 teaspoon garlic powder

Directions: Let the roast sit in room temperature for not less than 1 hour.

Preheat your oven to 375°F (190°C). In a small cup, mix the pepper, garlic powder and salt together. Put the roast onto the wire rack in the roasting pan, fat side facing up and rib side facing down. Massage the roast with the prepared seasoning. Put in preheated oven and let it roast for 1 hour. Switch off the oven and don't take out the roast.

Keep the oven door closed. Keep the roast inside the oven for 3 hours. Switch the oven back on at 375°F (190°C) temperature to reheat the roast 30-40 minutes before it's time to serve. The temperature inside the oven should not be less than 145°F (62°C). Take the roast out from the oven and let it sit for 10 minutes before slicing for serving.

FOOLPROOF ROSEMARY CHICKEN WINGS

Serv.: 2| **Prep.:** 20m | **Cook:** 40m

Ingredients:
- ✓ 1 1/2 pounds chicken wings, cut apart at joints, wing tips discarded
- ✓ 10 sprigs rosemary
- ✓ 1/2 whole head garlic, separated into cloves - cloves unpeeled and quartered
- ✓ 1 tablespoon olive oil, or as needed
- ✓ 1 teaspoon lemon pepper
- ✓ 1 teaspoon seasoned salt, or to taste

Directions: Turn the oven to 350°F (175°C) to preheat. On a broiler-proof baking sheet, place garlic cloves, rosemary, and chicken wings; ensure that they don't touch each other. Drizzle over the garlic and chicken with olive oil. Use seasoned salt and lemon pepper to season all sides of the wings. Bake for 35-40 minutes in the preheated oven until the juices run clear and around the bone of the chicken meat is not pink anymore, flipping the wings 1 time when they have cooked for 1/2 of the time. An instant-read thermometer should display a minimum of 160°F (70°C) when you insert it into the thickest sections of a wing.

Remove the baking sheet from the oven and turn the oven's broiler to High. Take the rosemary and garlic from the sheet and put aside. Flip the wings again.

Broil the wings for 5 minutes until turning golden brown. Use garlic and rosemary sprigs to garnish and enjoy.

July Salad

Serv.: 15 | **Prep.:** 10m | **Cook:** 0

Ingredients:
- ✓ 1 cup blueberries
- ✓ 1 cup sliced strawberries
- ✓ 1 cup chopped watermelon
- ✓ 1 cup red grapes
- ✓ 1 cup shredded coconut

Directions: In a bowl, combine grapes, watermelon, strawberries and blueberries then place in coconut.

Fragrant Lemon Chicken

Serv.: 6 | **Prep.:** 20m | **Cook:** 6-8h

Ingredients:
- ✓ 1 apple - peeled, cored and quartered
- ✓ 1 stalk celery with leaves, chopped
- ✓ 1 (3 pound) whole chicken
- ✓ Salt to taste
- ✓ Ground black pepper to taste
- ✓ 1 onion, chopped
- ✓ 1/2 teaspoon dried rosemary, crushed
- ✓ 1 lemon, zested and juiced
- ✓ 1 cup hot water

Directions: Rub pepper and salt on the skin of the chicken, then put celery and apple inside the chicken. Put the chicken in the slow cooker. Sprinkle chicken with lemon juice and zest, rosemary, and chopped onion. Add 1 cup of hot water into the slow cooker.
Cook, covered, on High for 1 hour. Change to low and cook for 6 to 8 hours, basting a few times.

Chopped Salsa

Serv.: 16 | **Prep.:** 25m | **Cook:** 0

Ingredients:
- ✓ 7 roma (plum) tomato, seeded and diced
- ✓ 6 cloves garlic, minced
- ✓ 6 jalapeno peppers, seeds and ribs removed, minced
- ✓ 1 small red onion, finely chopped
- ✓ 1 cup finely chopped cabbage
- ✓ 1 bunch fresh cilantro, chopped
- ✓ 1/3 cup fresh lime juice
- ✓ Salt to taste

Directions: In a big bowl, mix together lime juice, cilantro, cabbage, red onion, jalapenos, garlic and tomatoes. Season with salt to taste and chill for a couple of hours before serving.

Famous Spaghetti Sauce

Serv.: 8 | **Prep.:** 15m | **Cook:** 30m

Ingredients:
- ✓ 1 tablespoon olive oil
- ✓ 1 onion, chopped
- ✓ 1 green bell pepper, chopped
- ✓ 3 cloves garlic, minced
- ✓ 4 fresh mushrooms, sliced
- ✓ 1 pound ground turkey
- ✓ 1 pinch dried basil
- ✓ 1 pinch dried oregano
- ✓ Ground black pepper to taste
- ✓ 1 (14.5 ounce) can stewed tomatoes
- ✓ 2 (15 ounce) cans tomato sauce
- ✓ 1 (6 ounce) can tomato paste

Directions: The first part of this dish is simply sautéing garlic, green bell pepper, and onions together in olive oil in a big skillet over medium heat until the bell pepper is tender and onions are translucent. Put in the ground black pepper, oregano, basil, ground turkey, and mushrooms; fry while stirring frequently until the turkey is cooked. To the same pan you used for the first part, add the can of stewed tomatoes with the liquid. Lower the heat once you've added this and allow it to simmer until the tomatoes turn soft and start to fall apart. Put in tomato sauce and stir; thicken it by adding tomato paste. Turn the heat down to very low and allow the sauce to simmer for 15 minutes. Serve this with your preferred pasta.

French Fry Seasoning

Serv.: 5 | **Prep.:** 5m | **Cook:** 0

Ingredients:
- ✓ 2 teaspoons garlic salt
- ✓ 2 teaspoons onion salt
- ✓ 2 teaspoons salt
- ✓ 2 teaspoons ground paprika

Directions: In a bowl, mix together paprika, salt, onion salt and garlic salt. Turn into a zippered container to store.

French Canadian Gorton Pork Spread

Serv.: 16 | **Prep.:** 5m | **Cook:** 1h10m

Ingredients:
- ✓ 1 pound lean pork butt, cut into pieces
- ✓ 1 onion, chopped
- ✓ 1/2 teaspoon ground cinnamon
- ✓ 1/4 teaspoon ground cloves
- ✓ Salt and black pepper to taste

Directions: Get a saucepan then put the onion, cinnamon, pork and clove then add pepper and salt to taste. Add the water enough to cover meat. Turn on the stove to high heat, then minimize heat to medium-low and cover the saucepan for about 1 hour to cook until water has nearly absorbed. Occasionally stir to make the pork cook evenly. Make the pork into thin strands using a potato masher or wire whisk then remove the excess liquid and scoop out the gorton into a serving bowl. Place in the refrigerator until cold. Then serve.

Ginger Cabbage Patch Smoothie

Serv.: 2 | **Prep.:** 10m | **Cook:**

Ingredients:
- ✓ 1 cup roughly chopped cabbage
- ✓ 1 cup red grapes
- ✓ 1 red apple, cored and chopped
- ✓ 1 large carrot, peeled and chopped
- ✓ 1/2 cup water
- ✓ 1/2 cup ice cubes
- ✓ 1 tablespoon chopped fresh ginger

Directions: Combine carrot, ginger, grapes, cabbage, ice cubes, water, and apple in a blender. Blend until the mixture is smooth.

Ginger Sesame Salmon

Serv.: 4 | **Prep.:** | **Cook:** 20m

Ingredients:
- ✓ 4 thin onion slices, separated into rings
- ✓ 2 sheets (12x18-inches each) Reynolds Wrap® Non-Stick Foil
- ✓ 2 medium carrots, cut into julienne strips or shredded
- ✓ 4 (4 ounce) salmon fillets, thawed
- ✓ 2 teaspoons grated fresh ginger
- ✓ 2 tablespoons seasoned rice vinegar
- ✓ 1 teaspoon sesame oil
- ✓ Salt and pepper to taste
- ✓ Fresh spinach leaves

Directions: Set grill to medium-high heat or preheat oven to 450°F.
Place 1/4 of onion slices and carrots in the center of each sheet Reynolds Wrap® nonstick foil. Lay salmon atop vegetables. Scatter ginger over salmon; drizzle with oil and vinegar. Scatter pepper and salt on top to season.
Bring the foil sides up. Double fold ends and top to seal packet, leaving space for heat circulation inside. Do the same with the remaining foil, making 4 packets in total.
Bake in the preheated oven on a cookie sheet, 16 to 20 minutes.
Or, grill in a covered grill for 14 to 16 minutes.
Serve carrots and salmon over a bed of spinach. If desired, sprinkle top with extra seasoned rice vinegar.

GINGER AND LIME SALMON

Serv.: 6| **Prep.:** 15m | **Cook:** 15m

Ingredients:
- ✓ 1 (1 1/2-pound) salmon fillet
- ✓ 1 tablespoon olive oil
- ✓ 1 teaspoon seafood seasoning (such as Old Bay®)
- ✓ 1 teaspoon ground black pepper
- ✓ 1 (1 inch) piece fresh ginger root, peeled and thinly sliced
- ✓ 6 cloves garlic, minced
- ✓ 1 lime, thinly sliced

Directions: Position oven rack approximately 6 to 8 inches away from the heat source and preheat broiler; set oven's broiler to Low setting if there is. Line aluminum foil over a baking sheet.
Arrange salmon on the prepared baking sheet, skin side down; rub olive oil over the salmon. Season fish with black pepper and seafood seasoning. Place ginger slices on top of salmon and scatter garlic over. Arrange lime slices over ginger-garlic layer.
Broil salmon for about 10 minutes until heated through and starting to turn opaque; watch carefully. Turn broiler to high setting if there is; keep broiling for 5 to 10 minutes longer or until salmon is thoroughly cooked and easily flaked using a fork.

GLUTEN FREE SHAKE AND BAKE ALMOND CHICKEN

Serv.: 4| **Prep.:** 10m | **Cook:** 25m

Ingredients:
- ✓ 1/2 cup almond meal
- ✓ 1 teaspoon ground paprika
- ✓ 1 teaspoon sea salt
- ✓ 1 teaspoon ground black pepper
- ✓ 4 skinless, boneless chicken thighs

Directions: Preheat an oven to 175 °C or 350 °F. In a resealable bag, mix black pepper, sea salt, paprika and almond meal together. Into the bag, place every thigh of chicken, one by one; seal the bag and shake till equally coated. In glass baking dish, put the chicken.
In the prepped oven, bake for 25 minutes to half an hour till juices run clear and not pink anymore in the middle. An inserted instant-read thermometer into the middle should register at minimum of 74 °C or 165 °F.

GOAN PORK VINDALOO

Serv.: 8| **Prep.:** 30m | **Cook:** 1h25m

Ingredients:
- ✓ 16 dried Kashmiri chile peppers, stemmed and seeded
- ✓ 1 (1 inch) piece cinnamon stick
- ✓ 1 teaspoon cumin seeds
- ✓ 6 whole cloves
- ✓ 1/2 teaspoon whole black peppercorns
- ✓ 1/2 teaspoon ground turmeric
- ✓ 1 tablespoon white vinegar
- ✓ Salt to taste
- ✓ 2 pounds boneless pork loin roast, trimmed and cut into 1-inch cubes
- ✓ 1/4 cup vegetable oil
- ✓ 4 onions, chopped
- ✓ 10 cloves garlic, minced, or more to taste
- ✓ 1 (2 inch) piece fresh ginger root, minced
- ✓ 2 cups boiling water
- ✓ 2 green chile peppers, seeded and cut into strips
- ✓ 1/4 cup white vinegar

Directions: Using an electric coffee grinder or a mortar and pestle, grind turmeric, peppercorns, clove, cumin, cinnamon stick and Kashmiri chills till spices is smoothly ground. To make a smooth paste, combine with a tablespoon white vinegar. Season with salt to taste.
With the vinegar-spice paste, stir cubes of pork in a bowl till evenly coated. Put on plastic wrap to cover the bowl and refrigerate to marinate overnight.
In a big pot or Dutch oven, heat vegetable oil over medium-high heat. Cook and mix ginger, garlic, and onions for about 10 minutes, till golden brown. Put in the pork marinade and the pork, and cook for approximately 5 minutes, mixing often, till cubes of

pork have firmed. Add water, simmer, then lower the heat, place on the cover, and cook for about 40 minutes till pork is soft.

Mix in a quarter cup of vinegar and strips of green chile pepper. Cook without a cover for an additional of half an hour till vindaloo thickens and green chile peppers softens. Season with salt to taste prior to serving.

GOAN PRAWN PULAO

Serv.: 6 | **Prep.:** 10m | **Cook:** 20m

Ingredients:
- ✓ 1/2 pound prawns, peeled and deveined
- ✓ Sea salt to taste
- ✓ 1/2 cup grated coconut
- ✓ 4 Kashmiri chile peppers
- ✓ 1 tablespoon coriander seeds
- ✓ 3 cloves garlic, peeled
- ✓ 5 peppercorns
- ✓ 1 tablespoon vegetable oil
- ✓ 1 small onion, sliced
- ✓ 1/4 teaspoon ground turmeric
- ✓ 1 1/2 cups water, or as needed
- ✓ 3 ounces okra, cut into thirds
- ✓ 3 pieces kokum

Directions: Season prawns with sea salt.

Using a mortar and pestle to crush peppercorns, garlic, coriander seeds, chile peppers, and coconut together until the masala is evenly orange.

In a pot, heat oil over medium heat, stir and cook the onion for 5-10 minutes until slightly browned and tender. Stir turmeric and masala into the onion, cook for 1 minute until aromatic. Fill with enough water to create a creamy and substantial gravy.

Boil the gravy, add okra and prawns and cook for 10 minutes until the okra is soft and the prawns are heated through. Mix kokum in the prawn mixture and boil again. Take the pot away from the heat and let sit.

GOAT AND BUTTERNUT SQUASH STEW

Serv.: 4 | **Prep.:** 15m | **Cook:** 1h50m

Ingredients:
- ✓ 1 teaspoon ground cumin
- ✓ 1 teaspoon ground coriander
- ✓ 1 teaspoon ground ginger
- ✓ 1/2 teaspoon sweet paprika
- ✓ 1/2 teaspoon smoked sweet paprika
- ✓ 1/2 teaspoon smoked hot paprika
- ✓ 1/2 teaspoon ancho chile powder
- ✓ 1 (3 pound) bone-in goat shank
- ✓ 1/4 teaspoon salt, or more to taste
- ✓ 1/4 teaspoon ground black pepper, or to taste
- ✓ 2 tablespoons coconut oil
- ✓ 1 onion, chopped
- ✓ 1 (1 pound) butternut squash, peeled and cut into 1/2-inch cubes
- ✓ 4 cloves garlic, minced
- ✓ 1 (14 ounce) can diced tomatoes
- ✓ 1 1/2 cups water
- ✓ 1 cinnamon stick
- ✓ 1 pinch saffron

Directions: In a bowl, mix coriander, cumin, sweet paprika, ginger, smoked sweet paprika, chile powder and smoked hot paprika together.

Use about 1/4 teaspoon of pepper and 1/4 teaspoon of salt to rub goat shank.

In a large Dutch oven, heat coconut oil over medium-high heat until shimmering and melted. Cook goat shank in hot oil for around 2 to 3 minutes per side till browned as completely as you can get it. In a bowl, place shank, reserving oil in the skillet.

Set the heat of the skillet down to low heat. In the retained oil, cook and stir onion for approximately 7 to 10 minutes until softened. Add garlic and butternut squash; cook and stir for nearly 1 minute until the garlic is fragrant. Use the cumin mixture to sprinkle over the squash mixture; cook and stir for another 1 minute.

Into the squash mixture, mix water, tomatoes, saffron and cinnamon stick; place goat shank back to the Dutch oven, set the liquid to a simmer, and cook for about 90 minutes to 2 hours until the goat meat is falling from the bone and tender.

Take away shank from the Dutch oven then place to a cutting board. Strip meat from the bone and cut into pieces of bite-size. Discard bone. Blend meat into the squash mixture, add pepper and salt for seasoning, and cook for around 5 minutes until the meat is reheated.

GREEN SMOOTHIE

Serv.: 4 | **Prep.:** 10m | **Cook:** 0

Ingredients:
- ✓ 2 cups water
- ✓ 1 head romaine lettuce, chopped
- ✓ 1/2 cucumber, diced
- ✓ 1 avocado, peeled and pitted
- ✓ 2 stalks celery
- ✓ 2 ounces baby spinach leaves
- ✓ Lemon, juiced
- ✓ 2 cups ice
- ✓ 1 apple, cored
- ✓ 1 banana

Directions: In a blender, blend together spinach, water, lemon juice, romaine lettuce, avocado, cucumber and celery on high for about 30 seconds until smooth. Pour banana, apple and ice into the blender and then blend for about 30 seconds until smooth.

KOSHER DILLS

Serv.: 9 | **Prep.:** 15m | **Cook:** 20m

Ingredients:
- ✓ 3 cups water
- ✓ 1 cup distilled white vinegar
- ✓ 1/4 cup salt
- ✓ 2 cloves garlic, or more to taste
- ✓ 2 sprigs fresh dill, or more to taste
- ✓ 3 small cucumbers, or to taste
- ✓ 3 (1 pint) canning jars with lids and rings, or as needed

Directions: Boil salt, vinegar and water in a saucepan; cook for 2-3 minutes till salt melts. Sterilize the lids and jars for at least 5 minutes in boiling water. Pack garlic, dill and cucumbers in sterilized, hot jars. Put vinegar mixture over; fill to

within 1/4-in. from the top. Run a thin spatula/knife to remove any air bubbles around jar's insides after filling them. Use a moist paper towel to wipe the jar rims to remove any food residue. Put lids over; screw on rings.

Put a rack on the bottom of a big stockpot; use water to fill halfway. Boil; use a holder to lower the jars in boiling water, leave a 2-in. space between the jars. If needed, add more boiling water so water level is at least 1-in. above jar tops; put water on a rolling boil and cover the pot. Process for 15 minutes.

Take the jars from the stockpot; put on a wood/cloth-covered surface till cool, a few inches apart. Use a finger to press top of every lid when cool to be sure the seal is tight and lid doesn't move down or up at all; keep for 1 month minimum in a dark, cool area.

MEAT SAUCE

Serv.: 12 | **Prep.:** 15m | **Cook:** 2h45m

Ingredients:
- ✓ 1 tablespoon olive oil
- ✓ 1 pound sweet Italian sausage, sliced
- ✓ 1 pound round steak, cubed
- ✓ 1 pound veal, cubed
- ✓ 4 cloves garlic, chopped
- ✓ 2 (28 ounce) cans whole peeled tomatoes, crushed
- ✓ 1 tablespoon Italian seasoning
- ✓ 1 bay leaf
- ✓ 1/2 teaspoon garlic powder
- ✓ 1/2 teaspoon dried oregano
- ✓ 1/2 teaspoon ground black pepper
- ✓ 1/2 teaspoon dried parsley
- ✓ 1 (28 ounce) can tomato sauce

Directions: Heat olive oil in skillet on medium heat; cook veal, round steak and sausage till evenly browned for 10 minutes. Take meat from skillet; drain. Keep 1 tablespoon drippings. Mix garlic into skillet with reserved meat drippings; cook on medium heat for 3 minutes. Put crushed tomatoes in skillet; season with parsley, pepper, oregano, garlic powder, bay leaf and Italian seasoning. Cook for 15 minutes. Mix tomato sauce into skillet; cook for 15 minutes. Put meat in skillet. Lower heat to low; simmer for 2 hours, occasionally mixing.

GRAPEFRUIT SMOOTHIE

Serv.: 2| **Prep.:** 10m | **Cook:** 0

Ingredients:
- ✓ 3 grapefruit, peeled and sectioned
- ✓ 1 cup cold water
- ✓ 3 ounces fresh spinach
- ✓ 6 ice cubes
- ✓ 1 (1/2 inch) piece peeled fresh ginger
- ✓ 1 teaspoon flax seeds

Directions: Blend the ice cubes, flax seeds, water, grapefruit, ginger, and spinach in a blender or NutriBullet®, until the mixture is smooth.

GREEN DRAGON VEGGIE JUICE

Serv.: 1| **Prep.:** 5m | **Cook:** 0

Ingredients:
- ✓ 1/4 large lemon
- ✓ 1 cup fresh spinach, or to taste
- ✓ 2 sprigs fresh parsley, or more to taste
- ✓ 2 stalks celery
- ✓ 1/3 small jalapeno pepper (optional)
- ✓ 1 tomato, quartered
- ✓ 1 pinch salt
- ✓ 1 cup ice, or as desired

Directions: Process through a juicer with lemon, spinach, parsley, celery, jalapeno pepper and tomato, respectively. Season the juice with salt. Fill ice to a glass and pour juice into.

GREEN SLIME SMOOTHIE

Serv.: 4| **Prep.:** 5m | **Cook:** 0

Ingredients:
- ✓ 2 cups spinach
- ✓ 2 cups frozen strawberries
- ✓ 1 banana

- ✓ 2 tablespoons honey
- ✓ 1/2 cup ice

Directions: Freeze spinach for at least 1 hour until frozen. In a blender, mix ice, spinach, honey, strawberries, and banana together and blend until smooth. Serve immediately.

GREEN TOMATO AND BELL PEPPER DELIGHT

Serv.: 6| **Prep.:** 5m | **Cook:** 10m

Ingredients:
- ✓ 2 tablespoons olive oil
- ✓ 4 green tomatoes, chopped
- ✓ 1 green bell pepper, chopped
- ✓ 2 celery, chopped
- ✓ 1 bunch green onions, chopped
- ✓ 2 tablespoons apple cider vinegar

Directions: In a big skillet, heat the olive oil on medium heat. Stir in apple cider vinegar, green onions, celery, bell pepper and green tomatoes. Sauté for around 5-10 minutes until it becomes tender-crisp.

GRILLED AUBERGINES WITH PROSCIUTTO

Serv.: 2| **Prep.:** 10m | **Cook:** 7m

Ingredients:
- ✓ 1 eggplant, ends trimmed
- ✓ 1 red bell pepper, cut into rings and seeds removed
- ✓ 1 cup spinach leaves, torn into pieces
- ✓ 1 (1/2 ounce) slice thinly sliced prosciutto di Parma
- ✓ 1 teaspoon sun-dried tomato paste
- ✓ 1 tablespoon extra virgin olive oil
- ✓ 1 tablespoon balsamic vinegar
- ✓ 1/4 teaspoon dried oregano
- ✓ Freshly ground rock salt to taste

Directions: Set the oven's broiler to preheat to 200°C (400°F).

Place red bell pepper and eggplant slices on a baking tray. Broil for around 7 minutes for them to soften.

While waiting for the eggplant and pepper, add spinach to a serving plate and drizzle balsamic vinegar and olive oil over. Dust with salt for seasoning. When the vegetables are softened, place the red bell peppers over the spinach. Spread each eggplant slice with a small amount of sun-dried tomato paste. Add a slice of prosciutto on top. Place the eggplant slices on top of peppers to create an overlapping spiral pattern. Serve right away.

GRILLED BACON STUFFED STRAWBERRIES

Serv.: 10| **Prep.:** 5m | **Cook:** 5m

Ingredients:
- ✓ 10 fresh strawberries, hulled
- ✓ 4 slices cooked bacon, chopped

Directions: Preheat the grill to medium heat and grease the grill grate with a little bit of oil.

Use a paring knife to cut a small cone-shaped hollow at the top of each of the strawberries. Fill the hollow part of each strawberry with chopped bacon.

Put the bacon-filled strawberries on the preheated grill and let it cook for 2 minutes until it is hot, turn it often to evenly cook all sides.

GRILLED BEEF TENDERLOIN

Serv.: 13| **Prep.:** 30m | **Cook:** 55m

Ingredients:
- ✓ 1 (5 pound) whole beef tenderloin
- ✓ 6 tablespoons olive oil
- ✓ 8 large garlic cloves, minced
- ✓ 2 tablespoons minced fresh rosemary
- ✓ 1 tablespoon dried thyme leaves
- ✓ 2 tablespoons coarsely ground black pepper

- ✓ 1 tablespoon salt

Directions: To prepare the beef: Use a sharp knife to remove excess fat. For the thin tip end, fold under to about the thickness of the rest of the roast. Use butcher's twine to bind and continue to tie the roast with the twine every 1 1/2-2-in. (this can help the roast maintain its shape). Use scissors to snip the silver skin to make sure the roast does not bow while cooking. Combine salt, pepper, thyme, rosemary, garlic, and oil; rub this mixture over the roast until coated. Put the meat aside.

Set all gas burners on high for 10 minutes or build a charcoal fire in half the grill. Use tongs to lubricate the grate with a rag soaked with oil. On the hot rack, arrange the beef and grill, covered, for about 5 minutes until thoroughly seared. Flip the meat and grill, covered, for another 5 minutes until the second side has thoroughly seared.

Transfer the meat to the cool side of the charcoal grill, or turn off the burner directly beneath the meat and set the other 1 or 2 burners (depending on the grill style) to medium. Cook for 45-60 minutes until a meat thermometer reaches 130° for rosy pink when you insert one into the thickest part, depending on the grill and the size of the tenderloin. Allow the meat to sit for 15 minutes before carving.

GRILLED BEETS IN ROSEMARY VINEGAR

Serv.: 6| **Prep.:** 10m | **Cook:** 30m

Ingredients:
- ✓ 1/3 cup balsamic vinegar
- ✓ 1 teaspoon chopped fresh rosemary
- ✓ 1 clove garlic, peeled and crushed
- ✓ 1/2 teaspoon herbes de Provence
- ✓ 3 medium beets, sliced into rounds

Directions: Mix herbes de Provence, garlic, rosemary and balsamic vinegar in a medium bowl. Add beets in the mixture. Marinate for 20 minutes minimum.

Preheat outdoor grill to high heat; oil the grate lightly.

On a piece of foil, big enough to wrap all the ingredients, put the marinated mixture and beets; tightly seal. Put foil packet on the prepared grill. Cook till beets are tender for 25 minutes.
Take beets out of the packet. Put it on the grill grate directly for 2-5 minutes. Serve while hot.

GRILLED PORTOBELLO MUSHROOMS

Serv.: 3| **Prep.:** 10m | **Cook:** 10m

Ingredients:
- ✓ 3 portobello mushrooms
- ✓ 1/4 cup canola oil
- ✓ 3 tablespoons chopped onion
- ✓ 4 cloves garlic, minced
- ✓ 4 tablespoons balsamic vinegar

Directions: Clean mushrooms. Remove stems. Put aside for other use. On a plate, put caps, gill side up.
Mix vinegar, garlic, onion and oil in a small bowl. Evenly pour mixture on mushroom caps. Let it stand for an hour.
Grill for 10 minutes over hot grill. Immediately serve.

GRILLED SALMON WITH CURRIED PEACH SAUCE

Serv.: 2| **Prep.:** 15m | **Cook:** 15m

Ingredients:
- ✓ 2 fresh peaches, peeled and diced
- ✓ 1/4 cup honey
- ✓ 1 teaspoon curry powder
- ✓ Salt and pepper to taste
- ✓ 2 salmon steaks

Directions: Preheat the outdoor grill over medium-high heat and the coat grate lightly with oil.
Over medium heat, mix together the curry powder, honey, and peaches in a small saucepan. Heat to a simmer and then cook for about 10 minutes until the sauce becomes thick and peaches have broken down. Add pepper and salt to taste.

Season salmon steaks with pepper and salt and then cook for about 5 to 10 minutes on each side, depends on the thickness of the steaks, on the grill until fish easily flakes with a fork. Spread peach sauce atop salmon and serve.

GRILLED SAUSAGE STUFFED CALAMARI

Serv.: 8| **Prep.:** 20m | **Cook:** 15m

Ingredients:
- ✓ 2 tablespoons olive oil, divided, or as needed
- ✓ 1/2 cup diced onion
- ✓ 1/2 cup diced red bell pepper
- ✓ Salt and ground black pepper to taste
- ✓ 6 ounces spicy Italian sausage, removed from casings and crumbled
- ✓ 4 ounces calamari tentacles, minced
- ✓ 1/4 cup chopped fresh flat-leaf parsley
- ✓ 1 large egg
- ✓ 1/8 teaspoon smoked paprika
- ✓ 1 1/2 pounds cleaned calamari tubes
- ✓ 18 toothpicks, or as needed

Directions: In a skillet, heat 1 tablespoon olive oil on medium heat. Sauté red pepper and onion with a bit of salt in hot oil for 5-7 minutes until onion is translucent and soft. Take off heat. Cool to room temperature.
In a bowl, mix pepper, salt, smoked paprika, egg, parsley, onion mixture, minced tentacles, and sausage until evenly mixed. Place mixture in a piping bag.
Pipe the sausage mixture to tubes. Fill each tube to 2/3 full. On the top of every tube, thread a toothpick to fasten opening together. Put stuffed tubes onto a plate. Use plastic wrap to cover plate. Keep in fridge for about 1 hour to chill completely.
Heat an outdoor grill to medium-high heat. Oil grate lightly.
Brush leftover olive oil on tubes to coat all the sides. Season using salt.
On preheated grill, cook stuffed calamari for 10-12 minutes, occasionally turning, until stuffing is cooked through. An instant-read thermometer poked in the middle will say 68°C/155°F.

HAWKEYE PORK ROAST

Serv.: 10| **Prep.:** 5m | **Cook:** 1h30m

Ingredients:
- ✓ 1 (3 pound) boneless pork loin
- ✓ 2 tablespoons onion powder
- ✓ 2 tablespoons garlic powder
- ✓ 1 tablespoon ground black pepper

Directions: Turn the oven to 350°F (175°C) to preheat.
Use black pepper, garlic powder and onion powder to evenly season the pork loin; put in a roasting pan.
Cook for 90 minutes until the middle of the pork is not pink anymore. An instant-read thermometer should display 145°F (63°C) when you insert it into the middle.

HEALTHIER BAKED SLOW COOKER CHICKEN

Serv.: 6| **Prep.:** 25m | **Cook:** 8-10h

Ingredients:
- ✓ 1 (2 to 3 pound) whole chicken
- ✓ Salt and ground black pepper to taste
- ✓ 1 teaspoon paprika
- ✓ 3 large carrots, split lengthwise and cut into 2-inch pieces
- ✓ 2 medium onions, quartered
- ✓ 2 tablespoons fresh chopped parsley

Directions: Wad a piece of aluminum foil into 3- to 4-in. ball, working in the same manner to make 3 pieces; arrange them on the bottom of a slow cooker.
Rinse chicken under cold water, inside and out. Use paper towels to pat dry. Season paprika, pepper and salt on the chicken. Put the chicken into a slow cooker, on top of the crumbled aluminum foil.
Set the slow cooker on high for 1 hour; decrease to low for 4-5 hours. Add in vegetables; cook for around another 4-5 hours, or till the juices run

clear and the chicken is not pink anymore. Sprinkle parsley over. Serve.

HEALTHIER MARINATED GRILLED SHRIMP

Serv.: 6| **Prep.:** 15m | **Cook:** 6m

Ingredients:
- ✓ 3 cloves garlic, minced
- ✓ 2 tablespoons olive oil
- ✓ 1/4 cup tomato sauce
- ✓ 2 tablespoons red wine vinegar
- ✓ 2 tablespoons chopped fresh basil
- ✓ 1/2 teaspoon salt
- ✓ 1/4 teaspoon cayenne pepper
- ✓ 2 pounds fresh shrimp, peeled and deveined
- ✓ Skewers

Directions: In a large bowl, combine red wine vinegar, tomato sauce, olive oil and garlic. Use cayenne pepper, salt and basil for seasoning. Stir in shrimps until they are evenly coated. Put it in the refrigerator with cover, stirring one or two time, in 30 minutes or 1 hour.
Grease the grate lightly with oil; preheat the grill on medium heat.
Thread shrimps onto skewers, piercing once near head and once near tail. Throw away the marinate. Put the shrimps on the preheated grill and cook for 2 to 3 minutes per side until they turns opaque.

HEALTHIER TACO SEASONING

Serv.: 10| **Prep.:** 5m | **Cook:** 0

Ingredients:
- ✓ 1 clove garlic, peeled
- ✓ 1 teaspoon sea salt
- ✓ 1 tablespoon chili powder
- ✓ 1/4 teaspoon red pepper flakes
- ✓ 1/4 teaspoon dried oregano
- ✓ 1/2 teaspoon paprika
- ✓ 1 1/2 teaspoons ground cumin
- ✓ 1 teaspoon ground black pepper

Directions: Crush the garlic with salt until it forms

into a paste. In a small bowl, stir in pepper, cumin, paprika, oregano, red pepper flakes and chili powder. On the other hand, in a bowl of a mini food processor, mix together all the ingredients until well combined. Store it in the fridge in an airtight container.

HEALTHY LAMB MEATBALLS

Serv.: 4| **Prep.:** 20m | **Cook:** 30m

Ingredients:
- ✓ 1 pound ground lamb, or more to taste
- ✓ 1/2 cup shredded cabbage, or more to taste
- ✓ 1/3 cup diced onion
- ✓ 1 egg
- ✓ 1 1/4 tablespoons ground allspice
- ✓ 1 tablespoon freshly ground cardamom
- ✓ 1/4 teaspoon ground turmeric (optional)
- ✓ 1/4 teaspoon ground sumac (optional)
- ✓ Salt and ground black pepper to taste

Directions: Start preheating the oven at 350°F (175°C).
In a pot of water, heat lamb to a boil, crumbling into small chunks, using a spoon, until cooked completely, for 5 to 10 minutes. Discard fat from the water by a spoon and drain water from meat. Combine pepper, salt, sumac, turmeric, cardamom, allspice, egg, onion, cabbage, and cooked lamb in a bowl; roll to form into 1 1/2-inch balls.
Put meatballs on a baking sheet.
Bake in the prepared oven until meatballs are cooked thoroughly and turn brown on the outside, for 25 to 30 minutes.

HEARTY VENISON AND VEGETABLE BAKE

Serv.: 4| **Prep.:** 20m | **Cook:** 50m

Ingredients:
- ✓ 1 pound venison, cut into cubes
- ✓ 1 pound mushrooms, quartered
- ✓ 4 green onions, cut into 1/2-inch pieces
- ✓ 1 bulb fennel, sliced

- ✓ 2 parsnips, peeled and cut into 1/2 inch slices
- ✓ 2 tablespoons olive oil
- ✓ Salt and pepper to taste

Directions: Preheat an oven to 175 °C or 350 °F. In olive oil, toss parsnips, fennel, green onion, mushrooms and venison. Season with pepper and salt to taste; coat by tossing. Place onto a glass baking dish.
In prepped oven, bake for approximately 50 minutes till venison and vegetables are soft and browned.

HUNGARIAN GOULASH

Serv.: 8| **Prep.:** 15m | **Cook:** 2h

Ingredients:
- ✓ 1/3 cup vegetable oil
- ✓ 3 onions, sliced
- ✓ 2 tablespoons Hungarian sweet paprika
- ✓ 2 teaspoons salt
- ✓ 1/2 teaspoon ground black pepper
- ✓ 3 pounds beef stew meat, cut into 1 1/2 inch cubes
- ✓ 1 (6 ounce) can tomato paste
- ✓ 1 1/2 cups water
- ✓ 1 clove garlic, minced
- ✓ 1 teaspoon salt

Directions: On medium heat, heat oil in a Dutch oven or big pot; add onions. Cook and stir frequently until soft. Take out onions and let it stand.
Mix together pepper, 2 teaspoons of salt, and paprika in a medium bowl. Dredge beef cubes in the mixture. Cook beef cubes in the onion pot until all sides are brown. Place the onions back in the pot; add leftover a teaspoon of salt, tomato paste, garlic, and water. Turn heat to low and let it simmer, covered for 1 1/2 - 2 hrs until the beef is tender; stir from time to time.

HUNGARIAN HOT AND SPICY PICKLED CAULIFLOWER

Serv.: 39| **Prep.:** 20m | **Cook:** 10m

Ingredients:
- ✓ 4 cups distilled white vinegar
- ✓ 4 cups water
- ✓ 1/2 cup sea salt
- ✓ 1 head cauliflower, broken into florets
- ✓ 3 hot chile peppers, sliced lengthwise
- ✓ 3 cloves garlic, minced, divided
- ✓ 1 tablespoon mustard seed, divided
- ✓ 1 tablespoon whole black peppercorns, divided
- ✓ 1 tablespoon coriander seeds, divided
- ✓ 1 tablespoon dill seeds, divided
- ✓ 1 tablespoon allspice berries, divided
- ✓ 1 1/2 teaspoons red pepper flakes, divided
- ✓ 3 bay leaves
- ✓ 3 1-quart canning jars with lids and rings

Directions: In pot, mix salt, water and vinegar together; simmer.

In boiling water, sterilize lids and jars for a minimum of 5 minutes. Fill each jar with 1 bay leaf, half teaspoon red pepper flakes, a teaspoon allspice berries, a teaspoon dill seed, a teaspoon coriander seed, 1 teaspoon peppercorns, 1 teaspoon mustard seed, a minced garlic clove, a hot pepper and 1/3 cauliflower. Into jars, add vinegar mixture, filling to within half-inch of surface. Run a thin spatula or knife surrounding the inner of jars when filled to get rid of any air bubbles. Using moist paper towel, wipe jars rims to get rid of any food residue. Put lids on and screw on the rings.

In the base of a big stockpot, put a rack and fill with water midway. Boil and into boiling water, put down the jars with holder. Retain a 2 inches gap between jars. Put in additional boiling water if needed, for water level to reach at minimum of an-inch over the jar tops. Let water come to a rolling boil, put cover on pot, and process for 10 minutes. Take jars out of stockpot and put onto a wood or cloth-covered surface, a few inches away, till cool. When cool, push the surface of every lid using finger, making sure that seal is tight, lid should not move down or up at all. Keep in a dark, cool place.

HUNTER STYLE CHICKEN

Serv.: 4| **Prep.:** 15m | **Cook:** 40m

Ingredients:
- ✓ 4 tablespoons olive oil
- ✓ 1 (3 pound) whole chicken, cut into pieces
- ✓ 6 slices bacon, diced
- ✓ 2 onions, chopped
- ✓ 1 cup fresh sliced mushrooms
- ✓ 1 tablespoon chopped fresh parsley
- ✓ 1 tablespoon chopped fresh basil
- ✓ 1 teaspoon salt
- ✓ Freshly ground black pepper
- ✓ 1 cup white wine
- ✓ 1 pound tomatoes, diced

Directions: In a large skillet, heat oil; brown the chicken; remove. Add bacon; sauté for about 2 minutes over medium heat.

Add onions and mushrooms and keep sautéing until onions become translucent. Transfer chicken back to the skillet; scatter with pepper, salt, basil and parsley. Add tomatoes and wine. Simmer, covered, for 25-30 minutes; during cooking, turning the chicken once. Take the chicken out of the skillet; pour the sauce over the chicken.

HUNTER'S BEET CHIPS

Serv.: 4| **Prep.:** 15m | **Cook:** 30m

Ingredients:
- ✓ Cooking spray
- ✓ 5 large beets, peeled and thinly sliced
- ✓ 1 tablespoon olive oil, or as needed
- ✓ Salt and ground black pepper to taste

Directions: Prepare oven by heating it to 200° C or 400° F. Use cooking spray to grease a baking sheet. Arrange beets in one layer on the prepared baking sheet. Brush with olive oil on both sides of the beets. Add pepper and salt to taste.

Bake in oven for 15 minutes. Flip beets and cook for 15-20 minutes more until crisp. Move to wire rack and cool.

HURRICANE CARROTS

Serv.: 6| **Prep.:** 10m | **Cook:** 0

Ingredients:
- ✓ 1 cup shredded carrots
- ✓ 1 cup finely chopped apple
- ✓ 1/2 cup raisins
- ✓ 1/2 cup golden raisins
- ✓ 1 cup whole almonds
- ✓ 1/2 cup vegetable oil
- ✓ Salt and ground black pepper to taste

Directions: In a medium bowl, combine oil with almonds, all raisins, apple and carrots. Add pepper and salt for seasoning.

BREAKFAST SAUSAGE PATTIES

Serv.: 16| **Prep.:** 20m | **Cook:** 10m

Ingredients:
- ✓ 3 pounds ground pork
- ✓ 1 tablespoon molasses
- ✓ 1 tablespoon kosher salt
- ✓ 2 teaspoons ground black pepper, or to taste
- ✓ 1 1/2 teaspoons dried sage
- ✓ 1 1/2 teaspoons dried thyme
- ✓ 1 teaspoon red pepper flakes (optional)
- ✓ 1 teaspoon onion powder
- ✓ 1 teaspoon chopped fresh parsley
- ✓ 3/4 teaspoon ground nutmeg
- ✓ 1/2 teaspoon fennel seeds
- ✓ 1/2 teaspoon ground cayenne
- ✓ 1/2 teaspoon ground allspice

Directions: By hand, mix allspice, cayenne, fennel seeds, nutmeg, parsley, onion powder, red pepper flakes, thyme, sage, black pepper, salt, molasses and pork well in big bowl.
Divide the pork mixture to 16 portions; form into 1/4-in. thick patties.
Heat nonstick skillet on medium heat; in batches, pan-fry patties for 5 minutes per side till not pink in middle anymore and golden.

REAL MEXICAN CEVICHE

Serv.: 12| **Prep.:** 15m | **Cook:** 0

Ingredients:
- ✓ 4 pounds shrimp
- ✓ 1 pound scallops
- ✓ 6 large limes, juiced
- ✓ 1 large lemon, juiced
- ✓ 1 small white onion, chopped
- ✓ 1 cucumber, peeled and chopped
- ✓ 1 large tomato, coarsely chopped
- ✓ 1 jalapeno pepper, chopped
- ✓ 1 serrano pepper, chopped
- ✓ 1 bunch cilantro
- ✓ 1 tablespoon olive oil
- ✓ 1 tablespoon kosher salt
- ✓ Ground black pepper to taste

Directions: Toss the scallops and shrimp gently in a ceramic bowl or big glass with lemon juice and lime juice. Combine the pepper, salt, olive oil, cilantro, serrano, jalapeno, tomato, cucumber and onion. Cover the bowl and let the ceviche chill for an hour in the fridge, until the scallops and shrimp become opaque.

PORK CHORIZO

Serv.: 6| **Prep.:** 15m | **Cook:** 0

Ingredients:
- ✓ 2 pounds ground pork
- ✓ 2 teaspoons salt
- ✓ 4 tablespoons chili powder
- ✓ 1/4 teaspoon ground cloves
- ✓ 2 tablespoons paprika
- ✓ 2 cloves garlic, crushed
- ✓ 1 teaspoon dried oregano
- ✓ 3 1/2 tablespoons cider vinegar

Directions: Combine vinegar, oregano, garlic, paprika, ground cloves, chili powder, salt, and ground pork well. Put in an air-tight container to store in the fridge for the spices to combine before using, about 4 days.

JUMPING GINGER SMOOTHIE

Serv.: 1| **Prep.:** 15m | **Cook:** 0

Ingredients:
- ✓ 2 cups cold water
- ✓ 1 avocado, peeled, and pitted
- ✓ 1/2 cup fresh parsley
- ✓ 1 apple, cored and seeded
- ✓ 1 carrot, cut into chunks
- ✓ 1 lemon, peeled
- ✓ 1 leaf kale leaf, or more to taste
- ✓ 1 (1 inch) piece fresh ginger root, or more to taste
- ✓ 2 ice cubes (optional)
- ✓ 1 tablespoon flax seeds (optional)

Directions: Blend flax seeds, kale, apple, avocado, ice cubes, parsley, water, carrot, ginger, and lemon in a blender at high speed for 10-15 seconds until the mixture is smooth.

JUST PLAIN OL' CHILI

Serv.: 6| **Prep.:** 15m | **Cook: 2h45m**

Ingredients:
- ✓ 2 pounds lean ground beef
- ✓ 2 tablespoons olive oil
- ✓ 1 green bell pepper, diced
- ✓ 6 cloves garlic, minced
- ✓ 3 tablespoons ground cumin
- ✓ 1 tablespoon chili powder, or more to taste
- ✓ Salt and ground black pepper to taste
- ✓ 1 (28 ounce) can diced tomatoes
- ✓ 4 cups water

Directions: In a large skillet, heat over medium heat and add the ground beef; cook and stir until meat is not pink anymore, evenly browned, and crumbled, about 10 minutes. Discard all the excess grease.
Heat olive oil on medium-high heat in a soup pot. Cook and stir green pepper in the hot oil until it begins to soften, about 5 to 7 minutes. Lower the heat to low, blend in chili powder, cumin, and

garlic, and flavor with salt and black pepper to taste.
Combine cooked ground beef and tomatoes in the green bell pepper mixture, using a spatula to crumble tomatoes. Pour in 4 cups of water, or until enough to cover the ingredients, lower the heat to low, and simmer for at least 2 hours for the flavors to be well-blended.

KADHAI MURGH WITH BELL PEPPER

Serv.: 6| **Prep.:** 15m | **Cook:** 45m

Ingredients:
- ✓ 1 1/2 pounds skinless, boneless chicken breast, cut into bite-sized chunks
- ✓ 1/2 teaspoon salt
- ✓ 1/2 teaspoon ground turmeric
- ✓ 1/4 cup vegetable oil
- ✓ 2 onions, sliced thin
- ✓ 2 green bell peppers, cut into thin strips
- ✓ 4 green chile peppers, halved lengthwise
- ✓ 1/2 teaspoon cumin seed
- ✓ 1/2 teaspoon coriander seed
- ✓ 1/2 teaspoon whole black peppercorns
- ✓ 1/2 cinnamon stick
- ✓ 6 whole cloves
- ✓ 1 black cardamom pod
- ✓ 1/4 teaspoon fennel seed
- ✓ 1/2 cup water
- ✓ 2 tablespoons coconut milk powder
- ✓ 1/2 teaspoon ground red pepper
- ✓ Salt to taste
- ✓ 1/4 cup chopped fresh cilantro

Directions: Season the chicken evenly with turmeric and salt; put aside for 15 minutes.
In a kadhai or big skillet, heat oil over medium heat. In hot oil, let the onions cook for about 5 minutes till browned. Put in chicken and cook for an additional of approximately 5 minutes till browned. Into the chicken, mix chile peppers and bell peppers; keep cooking for 5 minutes more. Grind fennel seed, cardamom pod, cloves, cinnamon, black peppercorns, coriander seed and cumin seed into a coarse powder; scatter on top of mixture in the skillet. Put in salt, ground red

pepper, coconut milk powder and water. Cook for about half an hour till chicken is soft. Incase curry is too wet, cook on high till moisture evaporates. Jazz up with cilantro and serve while hot.

KALE CHIPS

Serv.: 2| **Prep.:** 15m | **Cook:** 35m

Ingredients:
- ✓ 1 bunch kale
- ✓ 1 tablespoon extra-virgin olive oil, divided
- ✓ 1 tablespoon sherry vinegar
- ✓ 1 pinch sea salt, to taste

Directions: Prepare oven by heating to 150° C or 300° F.
Remove inner ribs of each kale leaf and throw away. Tear the leaves evenly to pieces. (Usually about a size of a small potato chip when I make it.) Wash the leaves then dry using a salad spinner or with paper towels to completely remove water. Place kale pieces in a big resealable bag or a bowl if you want to use your hands. Place about half of the olive oil. Seal the bag and squeeze it so the oil coats kale evenly. Add the rest of the oil and squeeze the bag some more. Slightly "massage", making sure the oil evenly coats the leaves. Add the vinegar on kale leaves, seal the bag again, and shake to evenly distribute the vinegar on all the leaves. Arrange the leaves on a baking sheet evenly.
Roast in the oven for 35 minutes until almost crisp. Add salt to taste. Immediately serve.

PALEO ZUCCHINI CHIPS

Serv.: 6| **Prep.:** 15m | **Cook:** 45m

Ingredients:
- ✓ 1 tablespoon grated lime zest
- ✓ 2 teaspoons lime juice
- ✓ 2 teaspoons smoked paprika
- ✓ 1 teaspoon kosher salt
- ✓ 1/2 teaspoon ground black pepper
- ✓ 2 large zucchinis, thinly sliced
- ✓ Cooking spray

Directions: Heat oven to 110 degrees Celsius or 225 degrees Fahrenheit. Place parchment paper on a baking sheet.
Mix pepper, salt, paprika, lime juice, and lime zest in a bowl.
Put zucchini slices in one layer on the baking sheet. Grease using cooking spray then sprinkle lime mix on the top.
Bake in oven for 45-60 minutes until crispy and golden.

KOFTA KEBABS

Serv.: 28| **Prep.:** 45m | **Cook:** 5m

Ingredients:
- ✓ 4 cloves garlic, minced
- ✓ 1 teaspoon kosher salt
- ✓ 1 pound ground lamb
- ✓ 3 tablespoons grated onion
- ✓ 3 tablespoons chopped fresh parsley
- ✓ 1 tablespoon ground coriander
- ✓ 1 teaspoon ground cumin
- ✓ 1/2 tablespoon ground cinnamon
- ✓ 1/2 teaspoon ground allspice
- ✓ 1/4 teaspoon cayenne pepper
- ✓ 1/4 teaspoon ground ginger
- ✓ 1/4 teaspoon ground black pepper
- ✓ 28 bamboo skewers, soaked in water for 30 minutes

Directions: Use a mortar and pestle to mash garlic with salt until paste like. Use the flat side of the chef's knife and chopping board as an alternative way to create the paste. Stir garlic, onion, coriander, cumin, parsley, allspice, ginger, cayenne pepper, cinnamon, and pepper with lamb in a bowl. Stir mixture until well incorporated then mold in 28 balls. Make every ball around the tip of skewer and flat each into a 2-inch oval. Repeat with the rest of the skewers. On a baking sheet and transfer kebabs. For 30 minutes to 12 hours, refrigerate with cover.
Prepare the grill by lightly oiling the grate and preheat at medium heat.

Place the skewers on heated grill. Grill lamb while flipping occasionally until cooked to your desired doneness. For medium, grill 6 minutes.

KOREAN CUCUMBER SALAD

Serv.: 2| **Prep.:** 20m | **Cook:** 5m

Ingredients:
- ✓ 1/4 cup white vinegar
- ✓ 1/4 teaspoon black pepper
- ✓ 1/2 teaspoon red pepper flakes
- ✓ 1 teaspoon vegetable oil
- ✓ 2 tablespoons sesame seeds
- ✓ 1 cucumber, thinly sliced
- ✓ 1/2 green onion, sliced
- ✓ 1/2 carrot, julienned

Directions: Mix red pepper flakes, black pepper, and vinegar in a medium bowl.
In a saucepan, heat oil on medium-high heat. Mix in sesame seeds. Reduce the heat to medium. Cook for 5 minutes until seeds become brown. Take seeds out using a slotted spoon. Mix into the vinegar mixture. Stir in carrot, green onions, and cucumber. Cover then keep in fridge for at least five minutes.

SWEET POTATO FRIES

Serv.: 4| **Prep.:** 30m | **Cook:** 20m

Ingredients:
- ✓ 4 sweet potatoes, peeled and cut into long French fries
- ✓ 1/4 cup olive oil
- ✓ 1 teaspoon steak seasoning
- ✓ 1/2 teaspoon ground black pepper
- ✓ 1/2 teaspoon garlic powder
- ✓ 1/4 teaspoon salt
- ✓ 1/4 teaspoon paprika
- ✓ 1 tablespoon olive oil

Directions: In a big bowl, put sweet potato fries, sprinkle with a quarter cup olive oil, and coat by tossing. In another small bowl, combine paprika, salt, garlic powder, black pepper and steak seasoning till well mixed. Toss fries with olive oil using your left hand while drizzle the seasoning mixture over using right hand.
In a big skillet over medium heat, heat a tablespoon olive oil and put sweet potato pieces into the hot oil. Cover skillet and, pan-fry for 5 minutes; remove cover and flip fries. Put back cover over fries and cook for additional 5 minutes; keep flipping fries and covering for 10 minutes longer till sweet potatoes are soft.

LA GENOVESE

Serv.: 6| **Prep.:** 5m | **Cook:** 10m

Ingredients:
- ✓ 1/2 cup olive oil
- ✓ 1 pound lean ground beef
- ✓ 3 carrots, diced
- ✓ 1/2 onion, minced
- ✓ 1 teaspoon salt
- ✓ 1 pinch ground black pepper
- ✓ 3 tablespoons white wine

Directions: Put a large skillet over medium heat to heat olive oil. Add in beef; cook and stir well to break up clumps until it starts to brown. Add pepper, salt, onion and carrots; stir well. Cook for another 5 minutes with stirs until the meat extracts clear juice and the vegetables are just tender. Put in wine; continue cooking for another 1 minute and serve.

MANGO SALSA ON TILAPIA FILLETS

Serv.: 4| **Prep.:** 30m | **Cook:** 10m

Ingredients:
- ✓ 1/2 fresh pineapple - peeled, cored, and chopped
- ✓ 1/2 pound strawberries, quartered
- ✓ 3 kiwifruit, peeled and diced
- ✓ 1 large mango - peeled, seeded and diced
- ✓ 1/2 cup grape tomatoes
- ✓ 2 tablespoons finely chopped fresh cilantro
- ✓ 1 tablespoon balsamic vinegar
- ✓ 1 1/2 pounds tilapia fillets
- ✓ 1/2 teaspoon seasoned pepper blend

Directions: Add strawberries, mango, cilantro, tomatoes, pineapple, balsamic vinegar and kiwifruit in a bowl and toss it together.

Add a cooking spray in a pan and heat it over medium-high heat. Add seasoned pepper blend to the tilapia for seasoning and cook the fish in the frying pan for 2-3 minutes per side, until the fish turns opaque and white in color. Add the salsa on top of the fish before serving.

LAMB AND ASPARAGUS STEW

Serv.: 2| **Prep.:** 20m | **Cook:** 35m

Ingredients:
- ✓ 3 tablespoons vegetable oil
- ✓ 1 onion, chopped
- ✓ 1/2 pound cubed lamb stew meat
- ✓ 1/2 teaspoon salt
- ✓ 1/2 teaspoon ground black pepper
- ✓ 1 tablespoon ground turmeric
- ✓ 1/2 (6 ounce) can tomato paste
- ✓ 1 cup water
- ✓ 1 clove garlic, chopped
- ✓ 1 bunch fresh asparagus, trimmed and cut into 1 inch pieces

Directions: In a saucepan over medium high heat, heat vegetable oil. Stir in onions and cook for 2 minutes, remember to stir constantly while cooking. Add turmeric, pepper, salt and lamb; cook for about 3 minutes until the outside of lamb loses its pink color, remember to stir while cooking. Stir in garlic, water and tomato paste. Bring to a simmer, then lower the heat to medium-low, cover the saucepan and simmer for about 25 minutes until the lamb is softened.
When the lamb is soft, stir in asparagus and keep cooking for 3 minutes until asparagus is tender.

ROASTED SWEET POTATO BITES

Serv.: 1| **Prep.:** 10m | **Cook:** 20m

Ingredients:

- ✓ 1 cup peeled and cubed sweet potato
- ✓ 1/2 teaspoon coconut oil, melted
- ✓ 1 1/2 teaspoons chopped fresh rosemary
- ✓ 1 1/2 teaspoons chopped fresh thyme
- ✓ Salt and ground black pepper to taste

Directions: Set the oven to 190°C or 375°F.
In a bowl, add sweet potato cubes. Drizzle over potatoes with coconut oil and toss with your hands, until each cubes is coated. Spread the sweet potato cubes on a baking sheet, then season with pepper, salt, thyme and rosemary.
In the preheated oven, bake potatoes for approximately 20 minutes, until tender.

COCONUT FLAX MUG MUFFINS

Serv.: 1| **Prep.:** 5m | **Cook:** 1m

Ingredients:
- ✓ 1 egg
- ✓ 1/4 cup golden flaxseed meal
- ✓ 1 tablespoon unsweetened coconut flakes
- ✓ 1 teaspoon coconut oil
- ✓ 1 teaspoon unsweetened coconut milk beverage (such as Silk®)
- ✓ 1 teaspoon vanilla extract
- ✓ 1/2 teaspoon baking powder
- ✓ 1/2 teaspoon stevia powder

Directions: In a bowl, combine stevia, baking powder, vanilla extract, coconut beverage, coconut oil, coconut flakes, flaxseed meal and egg, then mix well. Place the batter into the microwave-safe mug. Cook for one minute on high in the microwave oven.

LOW CARB ZUCCHINI CHIPS

Serv.: 2| **Prep.:** 10m | **Cook:** 2h

Ingredients:
- ✓ 2 large large zucchini, thinly sliced
- ✓ 1 tablespoon olive oil, or to taste
- ✓ Sea salt to taste

Directions: Heat oven to 120 degrees Celsius or 250 degrees Fahrenheit.

Place the cut zucchini on the baking sheet. Lightly drizzle using olive oil and lightly sprinkle with some sea salt.

Bake in the oven for an hour on each side until they're like chips and entirely dry. Let it cool before eating.

Low Carb Zucchini Pasta

Serv.: 1| **Prep.:** 10m | **Cook:** 5m

Ingredients:
- ✓ 2 zucchinis, peeled
- ✓ 1 tablespoon olive oil
- ✓ 1/4 cup water
- ✓ Salt and ground black pepper to taste

Directions: Use a veggie peeler to cut zucchini lengthwise, stop when the seeds appear. Flip zucchini over and peel the rest of it into long strips; throw out seeds.

Slice zucchini strips into thinner threads that look like spaghetti.

In a big frying pan, heat olive oil on medium; cook the zucchini in the hot oil and stir, 1 minute. Add the water and cook 5-7 minutes until zucchini becomes soft. Use pepper and salt to season.

Quickie Chickie

Serv.: 2| **Prep.:** 10m | **Cook:** 10m

Ingredients:
- ✓ 2 teaspoons olive oil
- ✓ 6 ounces chicken tenderloin strips
- ✓ 1/4 teaspoon salt
- ✓ 1/8 teaspoon freshly ground black pepper
- ✓ 2 tablespoons chopped fresh basil
- ✓ 1 1/2 teaspoons honey
- ✓ 1 1/2 teaspoons balsamic vinegar, or more to taste

Directions: On medium-high heat, pour olive oil in a non-stick pan and heat. Sprinkle pepper and salt

on the chicken. Cook while regularly stirring the chicken in the hot oil for 3-5 minutes until it's not pink in the middle. Mix honey, balsamic vinegar, and basil into the chicken and stir Cook for another minute.

Magaricz

Serv.: 10| **Prep.:** 20m | **Cook:** 40m

Ingredients:
- ✓ 1/4 cup olive oil
- ✓ 1 large eggplant, peeled and coarsely chopped
- ✓ 1 medium red bell pepper, cut into thin strips
- ✓ 1 green bell pepper, cut into thin strips
- ✓ 1 large onion, diced
- ✓ 1 cup coarsely shredded carrot
- ✓ Salt to taste
- ✓ Crushed red pepper flakes

Directions: Lightly salt eggplant and place in a colander. Set aside for about 45 minutes, allowing eggplant to drain.

Heat olive oil in a big pan over medium high heat. Toss in eggplant, onion, carrot, red and green bell peppers.

Mix well to coat then turn heat down to low.

Continue cooking for 40 minutes, stirring from time to time, until mixture achieves coarse jam consistency. Sprinkle with salt and red pepper flakes to taste.

Refrigerate, covered, for at least 1 hour. Serve chilled with your preferred crackers or bread.

Mango Chutney

Serv.: 32| **Prep.:** 40m | **Cook:** 35m

Ingredients:
- ✓ 4 cups green (under ripe) mangoes - peeled, seeded, and diced
- ✓ 1/2 cup raisins
- ✓ 1/4 cup serrano peppers, finely chopped
- ✓ 6 cloves garlic, minced
- ✓ 1 1/2 tablespoons minced fresh ginger root

- ✓ 1 1/2 teaspoons lemon zest
- ✓ 1 tablespoon black pepper
- ✓ 2 tablespoons molasses
- ✓ 1 small cinnamon stick
- ✓ 4 whole cloves
- ✓ 1 cup water
- ✓ 1 cup cider vinegar

Directions: In a large saucepan, place cloves, cinnamon, molasses, black pepper, lemon zest, ginger, garlic, serrano peppers, raisins and mango. Transfer in vinegar and water.

Boil the mixture; turn the heat down to medium-low and simmer without a cover for around 30 minutes, or till it reaches a jam-like consistency. Mix frequently while cooking.

Allow to cool when thickened; place in a refrigerator for storage. You can also freeze the chutney.

MAPLE GLAZED BUTTERNUT SQUASH

Serv.: 4| **Prep.:** 10m | **Cook:** 20m

Ingredients:
- ✓ 1 butternut squash - peeled, seeded, quartered, and cut into 1/2-inch slices
- ✓ 2/3 cup water
- ✓ 1/4 cup maple syrup
- ✓ 1/4 cup dark rum
- ✓ 1/4 teaspoon ground nutmeg

Directions: Boil nutmeg, butternut squash, rum, maple syrup, and water together in a pot. Lower heat; let it simmer for 15m while stirring occasionally until the squash is tender.

With a slotted spoon move the butternut squash to a serving dish; save the liquid in the pot. Simmer for 5-10m until the liquid is thick and reduced; pour all over the butternut squash.

MAPLE GLAZED CHICKEN WITH SWEET POTATOES

Serv.: 4| **Prep.:** 15m | **Cook:** 30m

Ingredients:

- ✓ 1 1/2 pounds sweet potatoes, peeled and cut into 1-inch pieces
- ✓ 1 pound chicken tenders
- ✓ 2 teaspoons steak seasoning (such as Montreal Steak Seasoning®)
- ✓ 2 tablespoons vegetable oil
- ✓ 1/2 cup maple syrup
- ✓ 1/2 cup sliced green onions

Directions: Put the sweet potatoes into a large pot and add water to cover. Bring to a boil over high heat, then lower the heat to medium-low, and simmer for about 20 minutes, covered, until softened.

Drain and let them steam dry for a minute or two. Mash the potatoes and put aside.

Dust steak seasoning over chicken tenders; put oil in a large skillet and heat over medium heat, then add the chicken tenders and cook for 5-8 minutes each side, until the meat is not pink anymore inside and lightly browned.

Take off the chicken, and put aside Whisk maple syrup into the skillet, scraping up and dissolving any browned flavor bits from the skillet. Bring to a boil, simmer for 2 minutes, and mix in the green onions.

Put the mashed sweet potatoes onto a serving platter with chicken tenders on top and pour maple sauce over the chicken to serve.

MAPLE GLAZED SWEET POTATOES WITH BACON & CARAMELIZED ONIONS

Serv.: 12| **Prep.:** 30m | **Cook:** 1h5m

Ingredients:
- ✓ 4 pounds sweet potatoes, peeled and cut in 1-inch chunks
- ✓ 2 tablespoons olive oil
- ✓ 1 teaspoon salt
- ✓ 1/2 teaspoon ground black pepper
- ✓ 5 slices smoked bacon, chopped
- ✓ 1 pound onions, thinly sliced
- ✓ 1 cup pure maple syrup
- ✓ 2 teaspoons fresh thyme

Directions: Preheat an oven to 220 °C or 425 °F. In

a big bowl, toss black pepper, salt, olive oil and sweet potato chunks. On a big rimmed baking sheet, arrange the sweet potatoes.

In the prepped oven, roast for 40 minutes till soft and browned; mix after the initial 20 minutes. In a big skillet over medium heat, cook the bacon for 10 minutes till brown and crisp; put the bacon into a bowl, but retain grease in the skillet. In bacon grease, cook onions for 10 minutes till browned, mixing often. Turn heat down to low, and cook the onions for 10 to 15 minutes more till really tender, sweet and brown. Mix frequently. Blend onions with bacon in the bowl, and reserve. In the hot skillet, put maple syrup with thyme, and bring to a rolling boil. Boil syrup for 3 to 4 minutes till reduced by half. Put in onion-bacon mixture and roasted sweet potatoes, coat vegetables with maple glaze by mixing. Place into a serving dish.

MARINATED GRILLED SHRIMP

Serv.: 6| **Prep.:** 15m | **Cook:** 6m

Ingredients:
- ✓ 3 cloves garlic, minced
- ✓ 1/3 cup olive oil
- ✓ 1/4 cup tomato sauce
- ✓ 2 tablespoons red wine vinegar
- ✓ 2 tablespoons chopped fresh basil
- ✓ 1/2 teaspoon salt
- ✓ 1/4 teaspoon cayenne pepper
- ✓ 2 pounds fresh shrimp, peeled and deveined
- ✓ Skewers

Directions: Mix together red wine vinegar, tomato sauce, olive oil, and garlic in a large bowl. Sprinkle with salt, cayenne pepper, and basil. Put in the shrimps and stir to coat. Cover and refrigerate for half up to a full hour, stirring occasionally.
Preheat grill at medium. Skewer the shrimps, impaling near the tail and coming out near the head. Discard its marinade.
Lightly grease the grate. Grill for 2 to 3 minutes each side or until flesh is opaque.

MARINATED KEBABS

Serv.: 4| **Prep.:** 40m| **Cook:** 10m

Ingredients:
- ✓ 2 pounds premium meat
- ✓ 2 bell peppers (color of your choice)
- ✓ 1 onion
- ✓ 1/4 teaspoon dried thyme
- ✓ Salt and pepper
- ✓ 3 tablespoons olive oil
- ✓ 1 jar Maille® Dijon Originale Mustard
- ✓ Skewers

Directions: Slice the meat, onions, and bell peppers into squares.
Whisk together the contents of a jar of Maille® Dijon Originale mustard, thyme, olive oil, and salt and pepper in a large bowl. Toss in the meat to coat and marinate in the refrigerator for half an hour. Cue the meat alternately with the onions and the bell peppers onto skewers. Flip and baste frequently with remaining mixture while grilling.

CLAM CHOWDER

Serv.: 12| **Prep.:** 15m | **Cook:** 45m

Ingredients:
- ✓ 8 slices bacon
- ✓ 1 cup chopped onion
- ✓ 1 cup chopped celery
- ✓ 7 cups clam juice
- ✓ 3 (28 ounce) cans stewed tomatoes
- ✓ 5 tablespoons dried thyme
- ✓ 2 (6.5 ounce) cans minced clams

Directions: On medium heat, fry the bacon in a large saucepan until the meat turns crisp. Until done, remove from the pot and crush. In the same pot, cook the onion and celery until the onion turns translucent. Add in the tomatoes and clam juice. Season the mixture with thyme and then mix in the clams. Let simmer for 45 minutes for the flavors to blend well together.

MARINATED MUSHROOMS

Serv.: 8| **Prep.:** 10m | **Cook:** 0

Ingredients:
- ✓ 1 1/2 teaspoons garlic salt
- ✓ 1 1/2 teaspoons seasoning salt
- ✓ 1/4 cup distilled white vinegar
- ✓ 1/2 cup olive oil
- ✓ 2 (8 ounce) cans mushrooms, drained

Directions: Whisk the olive oil, vinegar, seasoned salt and garlic salt together. Spread over mushrooms and let marinate for 24 hours.

BAKED ONIONS

Serv.: 6| **Prep.:** 1h | **Cook:** 30m

Ingredients:
- ✓ 6 sweet onions
- ✓ 1/4 cup balsamic vinegar
- ✓ 1/4 cup honey
- ✓ 1/8 teaspoon fresh chopped tarragon

Directions: Set the oven to 175°C or 350°F to preheat.
Peel onions and form 2 cross slices on the surface of the onion. Put in a casserole dish or clay cooker. Combine tarragon, honey and balsamic vinegar together. Drizzle over onions and marinate about an hour.
Bake until onions are softened, or for about 30-40 minutes.

GRILLED FISH

Serv.: 4| **Prep.:** 10m | **Cook:** 10m

Ingredients:
- ✓ 1/4 cup olive oil
- ✓ 1 tablespoon dried parsley
- ✓ 2 tablespoons dried thyme
- ✓ 1 tablespoon dried rosemary
- ✓ 1 clove garlic, minced
- ✓ 4 (6 ounce) fillets salmon
- ✓ 1 lemon, juiced

Directions: Prepare the grill by preheating to medium heat.
Combine the garlic, rosemary, thyme, parsley, and olive oil in a shallow glass dish. Add the salmon in the dish, flipping to coat. Squeeze lemon juice over each fillet. Cover and refrigerate for 30 minutes to marinate.
Put oil lightly on the grill grate. Place salmon on the grill and get rid of any left marinade. Cook salmon on the preheated grill for 8-10 minutes over medium heat, flipping once. Fish is cooked once it flakes easily using a fork.

LAMB WITH SHIRAZ HONEY SAUCE

Serv.: 4| **Prep.:** 20m | **Cook:** 30m

Ingredients:
- ✓ 1 (7 bone) rack of lamb, trimmed and frenched
- ✓ Sea salt to taste
- ✓ 2 1/2 tablespoons ras el hanout
- ✓ 1 cup Shiraz wine
- ✓ 1/3 cup honey

Directions: Set the oven to 400°F (200°C) and start preheating.
Season lamb with sea salt; rub ras el hanout over it. Sear lamb on all sides in a medium cast iron skillet over medium-high heat until evenly browned.
Put the skillet with lamb in the prepared oven; roast for half an hour or until the internal temperature reached 145°F (63°C) as the minimum.
Take the lamb out of the skillet; reserve the juices; let stand for 10-15 minutes before you slice the ribs. Put the skillet with juices over medium heat; stir in honey and wine. Cook until the liquid reduces by about 1/2. Drizzle over ribs; serve.

SPICY CARROT SALAD

Serv.: 6| **Prep.:** 15m | **Cook:** 20m

Ingredients:

- ✓ 1 pound carrots, peeled and sliced into thin rounds
- ✓ 2 cups water
- ✓ 2 cloves garlic, minced
- ✓ 2 tablespoons olive oil
- ✓ 1/2 teaspoon sweet paprika
- ✓ 1 pinch cayenne pepper, or to taste
- ✓ Salt and ground black pepper to taste
- ✓ 1 tablespoon wine vinegar
- ✓ 1/2 teaspoon ground cumin
- ✓ 1/4 cup cilantro leaves

Directions: On medium-high heat, boil water, black pepper, carrots, salt, garlic, cayenne pepper, paprika, and olive oil together in a shallow pan for 20m until the water evaporates and the carrots are tender.
Mix cumin and vinegar into the carrot mixture.
Take off pan from heat then let set aside and let the mixture cool to room temperature.
Add cilantro on top then serve.

MURPHY STEAKS

Serv.: 4| **Prep.:** 30m | **Cook:** 10m

Ingredients:
- ✓ 2 pounds beef tenderloin steaks
- ✓ 1 bulb garlic, cloves separated and peeled
- ✓ Salt to taste
- ✓ Ground black pepper to taste

Directions: Remove garlic clove from the bulb and peel, then cut into strips lengthwise.
Punch holes into steak using a sharp knife, then stuff garlic strips into holes. Cover and put it in the refrigerator for at least 4 hours.
Preheat grill to hot heat.
Oil the grate lightly. Put the steaks stuffed with garlic on hot grill with garlic stuff up. Cook for 4 to 5 minutes. Turn and use pepper and salt to season. Continue cooking for another 4 to 5 minutes until done.

MUSHROOMS AND SPINACH ITALIAN STYLE

Serv.: 4| **Prep.:** 20m | **Cook:** 10m

Ingredients:
- ✓ 4 tablespoons olive oil
- ✓ 1 small onion, chopped
- ✓ 2 cloves garlic, chopped
- ✓ 14 ounces fresh mushrooms, sliced
- ✓ 10 ounces clean fresh spinach, roughly chopped
- ✓ 2 tablespoons balsamic vinegar
- ✓ 1/2 cup white wine
- ✓ Salt and freshly ground black pepper to taste
- ✓ Chopped fresh parsley, for garnish

Directions: In a big skillet, heat olive oil on moderately high heat. Sauté garlic and onion in the oil until they begin to soften.
Put in mushrooms and fry for 3-4 minutes, until they start to shrink. Toss in the spinach and fry until wilted, while stirring continuously, or for a several minutes.
Put in vinegar while stirring continuously until it is absorbed, then stir in white wine. Lower heat to low and simmer until the wine has nearly fully absorbed.
Season to taste with pepper and salt, then sprinkle over with fresh parsley. Serve hot.

MUSSELS IN A FENNEL AND WHITE WINE BROTH

Serv.: 4| **Prep.:** 10m | **Cook:** 45m

Ingredients:
- ✓ 1 tablespoon olive oil
- ✓ 1 bulb fennel, trimmed and thickly sliced
- ✓ 1 1/2 tablespoons olive oil
- ✓ 3 cloves garlic, thinly sliced
- ✓ 1 pound mussels, cleaned and debearded
- ✓ 1 cup halved cherry tomatoes
- ✓ 1/2 cup white wine
- ✓ 1/4 cup chopped fresh flat-leaf parsley

Directions: Start heating oven to 400 deg F or 200 deg C. Put a silicone baking mat or parchment paper on a baking sheet to line.

Put fennel slices in a bowl. Over fennel, add 1 tablespoon olive oil and mix to coat. Put on the prepared baking sheet, then into the heated oven, roast for 25 to 35 minutes until fennel is heated through and becoming caramelize.

Over medium-high temperature, heat 1 1/2 tablespoons olive oil in a large skillet. Put in garlic and cook 1 to 2 minutes. Stir frequently until garlic becomes fragrant and turns light golden in color. Add mussels to garlic and toss to evenly mix. Pour in cherry tomatoes, roasted fennel, and white wine. Heat to a boil, put lid on, and cook for 3 to 5 minutes or until mussels open. Mix parsley in and serve.

GOULASH

Serv.: 6 | **Prep.:** 25m | **Cook:** 35m

Ingredients:
- ✓ 1 pound lean ground beef
- ✓ 1 (8 ounce) package fresh mushrooms, sliced
- ✓ 1 green bell pepper, cut into 1/2 inch pieces
- ✓ 1 red bell pepper, cut into 1/2 inch pieces
- ✓ 1 zucchini, thickly sliced
- ✓ 1 small red onion, sliced
- ✓ 4 tablespoons olive oil
- ✓ 1/2 tablespoon paprika
- ✓ 1/2 tablespoon dried basil
- ✓ 1 teaspoon garlic salt
- ✓ 1/2 teaspoon white pepper
- ✓ 1 (14.5 ounce) can whole peeled tomatoes with liquid, chopped

Directions: Brown ground beef in a big frying pan. Take the beef out using a slotted spoon and remove the fat.

Put the frying pan into the stove again. Add in olive oil and heat over medium-high heat. Mix in pepper, garlic salt, basil, paprika, onion, squash, red and green peppers, and mushrooms. Cook for 5 minutes, you can stir it occasionally.

Lower the heat to medium. Mix in tomatoes and beef; simmer for 20 minutes, you stir it occasionally.

NETTLES

Serv.: 4 | **Prep.:** 10m | **Cook:** 7m

Ingredients:
- ✓ 1/2 cup olive oil
- ✓ 1/3 cup water
- ✓ 5 cloves garlic, minced
- ✓ 5 cups nettle leaves, stalks trimmed off
- ✓ Salt and ground black pepper to taste

Directions: In a big skillet, heat olive oil with water on medium heat. Put in garlic, then simmer for approximately 2 minutes until aromatic. Lower the heat slightly and blend in nettle leaves with a wooden spoon. Cook for around 5 minutes while stirring frequently, until leaves are softened and emerald green in color. Season with pepper and salt.

NO TOMATO PASTA SAUCE

Serv.: 8 | **Prep.:** 5m | **Cook:** 45m

Ingredients:
- ✓ 2 (15 ounce) cans sliced carrots, drained
- ✓ 1 (15 ounce) can sliced beets, drained
- ✓ 1 tablespoon olive oil
- ✓ 4 cloves garlic, minced
- ✓ 1 onion, chopped
- ✓ 1 bay leaf
- ✓ 2 tablespoons Italian seasoning
- ✓ 1/4 cup red wine vinegar

Directions: One can at a time, put beets and carrots in blender; blend till smooth. In skillet, heat olive oil on medium heat; mix and cook onions and garlic till onions are translucent. Mix pureed beets and carrots in; add red wine vinegar, Italian seasoning and bay leaf. Cover; cook till sauce starts to boil. Remove lid; lower heat to low. Simmer for at least 30 minutes or for up to 4 hours.

TOMATO FREE MARINARA SAUCE

Serv.: 2| **Prep.:** 25m | **Cook:** 32m

Ingredients:
- ✓ 1/4 kabocha squash, peeled and cut into small cubes
- ✓ 3 carrots, cut into small cubes
- ✓ 1/2 red beet, cut into small cubes
- ✓ 1 1/2 teaspoons olive oil
- ✓ 1/3 yellow onion, finely chopped
- ✓ 1 clove garlic, minced
- ✓ 5 leaves fresh sage, finely chopped
- ✓ 1 tablespoon capers (optional)
- ✓ 1 tablespoon dried Italian herbs
- ✓ 1 pinch Himalayan salt to taste
- ✓ 1/2 cup water, or more if needed
- ✓ 1/2 lemon, juiced
- ✓ 5 leaves fresh basil, chopped

Directions: In food processor, mix beet, carrots and kabocha squash; pulse till roughly grated.
In a saucepan, heat olive oil till sizzling over medium heat. Put in sage, garlic and onion; cook and mix for a minute, or till onion is aromatic. Mix in salt, Italian herbs, capers and grated kabocha squash mixture.
In the saucepan, put the water. Place cover on and let sauce simmer for half an hour, putting additional water if necessary, or till kabocha squash mixture is tender. Using a fork, crush mixture to create a smoother sauce.
Mix basil and lemon juice into sauce and allow the flavors to blend for a minute.

NORI CHIPS

Serv.: 2| **Prep.:** 5m | **Cook:** 5m

Ingredients:
- ✓ 1 sheet nori (dried seaweed), cut into thin strips
- ✓ 1 teaspoon olive oil, or as needed
- ✓ Salt to taste

Directions: Start preheating oven to 150 degrees C (300 degrees F). Spray baking sheet lightly with oil.

On the prepared baking sheet, place nori smooth-side down. Lightly brush nori with olive oil; add salt.
In the preheated oven, bake for 3 to 4 minutes until nori is dry and crispy.

AVOCADO & PISTACHIOS

Serv.: 2| **Prep.:** 10m | **Cook:** 0

Ingredients:
- ✓ 1 tablespoon shelled pistachios
- ✓ 1 tablespoon almonds
- ✓ 3/4 cup unsweetened coconut milk
- ✓ 5 cubes ice cubes
- ✓ 1/2 large avocado, peeled and pitted
- ✓ 1 tablespoon honey
- ✓ 1 pinch saffron threads (optional)

Directions: In a blender, blend almonds and pistachios until ground; put in saffron, honey avocado, ice cubes, and coconut milk. Blend until smooth.

PALEO KALE CHIPS

Serv.: 4| **Prep.:** 5m | **Cook:** 20m

Ingredients:
- ✓ Olive oil cooking spray
- ✓ 1 bunch kale, ribs removed and leaves torn into pieces
- ✓ 1 tablespoon coconut oil
- ✓ 1 pinch garlic salt, or to taste
- ✓ Salt and ground black pepper to taste

Directions: Heat oven to 230 degrees Celsius or 450 degrees Fahrenheit. Use cooking spray to grease a baking sheet.
Place kale and coconut oil in a bowl. Toss using your hands until coated. Place the kale on the baking sheet. Sprinkle pepper, salt, and garlic salt on top of the kale.
Put baking sheet in the oven and turn it off. Place the kale for 20 minutes in the oven until crisp.

PALEO MAPLE BACON MINI DONUTS

Serv.: 13| **Prep.:** 20m | **Cook:** 14m

Ingredients:
- ✓ 3 slices bacon, or more to taste
- ✓ 1 cup cassava flour (such as Otto's)
- ✓ 1 teaspoon baking powder
- ✓ 1/4 teaspoon salt
- ✓ 1/4 cup butter, at room temperature
- ✓ 2 tablespoons coconut sugar
- ✓ 3/4 cup coconut milk, at room temperature
- ✓ 1/4 cup maple syrup, at room temperature
- ✓ 1 egg, at room temperature
- ✓ 1/2 teaspoon vanilla extract
- ✓ Topping:
- ✓ 6 tablespoons almond butter, at room temperature
- ✓ 3 tablespoons maple syrup, at room temperature
- ✓ 2 tablespoons coconut milk, at room temperature (optional)

Directions: Put bacon in a big skillet and cook on medium-high heat for 10 minutes and turn occasionally or until it's evenly browned. Use paper towels to drain bacon slices. Reserve the bacon drippings in the skillet. Chop the bacon.
Mix salt, baking powder, and cassava flour in a bowl.
Mix coconut sugar and butter with an electric mixer in a bowl until fluffy. Add egg, 1/4 cup of maple syrup, and 3/4 cup of coconut milk mix until fully combined. Mix the flour mix in butter mix until you get a smooth batter. Place in 1 tablespoon of bacon drippings at a time if the batter is very thick. Place chopped bacon in the batter.
Heat the donut maker following the manufacturer's instructions.
Move batter into a clear plastic bag and cut off a corner. Fill the donut maker with the batter following the instructions of the manufacturer.
Cook it for 4-5 minutes. Place the donuts on a wire rack. Let cool for 15 minutes.
Mix 2 tablespoons of coconut milk, 3 tablespoons of maple syrup, and almond butter in a bowl until it's extremely smooth. Dip the cooled donuts in the almond butter topping.

PALEO PEACH CRISP WITH COCONUT AND SLIVERED ALMONDS

Serv.: 4| **Prep.:** 10m | **Cook:** 30

Ingredients:
- ✓ 1 (16 ounce) package frozen peach slices
- ✓ 2 tablespoons coconut sugar, divided
- ✓ 1 1/2 cups almond flour
- ✓ 1/2 cup coconut flakes
- ✓ 1 teaspoon baking powder
- ✓ 1/2 teaspoon sea salt
- ✓ 3 tablespoons unsalted butter, cubed
- ✓ 1 teaspoon vanilla extract
- ✓ 1/4 cup slivered almonds
- ✓ 1 tablespoon coconut oil, melted

Directions: Preheat an oven to 175 °C or 350 °F. In baking dish, put slices of peach.
In preheating oven, defrost the peaches for 5 minutes. Separate and scatter equally in baking dish. Scatter a tablespoon of sugar over.
In food processor, mix salt, baking powder, coconut flakes, almond flour and leftover 1 tablespoon of coconut sugar; pulse approximately five times till blended. Put the vanilla extract and butter; pulse several more times till crumbly. Put on top of peaches.
On top of flour mixture, spread slivered almonds. Drizzle top with coconut oil.
In prepped oven, bake for 22 to 25 minutes till golden brown.

PALEO PECAN MAPLE SALMON

Serv.: 4| **Prep.:** 15m | **Cook:** 15m

Ingredients:
- ✓ 4 (4 ounce) fillets salmon
- ✓ Salt and ground black pepper to taste
- ✓ 1/2 cup pecans
- ✓ 3 tablespoons pure maple syrup
- ✓ 1 tablespoon apple cider vinegar

- ✓ 1 teaspoon smoked paprika
- ✓ 1/2 teaspoon chipotle pepper powder
- ✓ 1/2 teaspoon onion powder

Directions: On a baking sheet, put salmon fillets. Use black pepper and salt to season.
In a food processor, mix together onion powder, chipotle powder, paprika, vinegar, maple syrup, and pecans, pulse until the mixture is powdery. Put the pecan mixture on top of each salmon fillet, fully cover the entire surface. Chill the covered salmon for 2-3 hours do not put a cover on.
Start preheating the oven to 425°F (220°c).
Put the salmon in the preheated oven and bake for 12-14 minutes until a fork can easily flake the fish.

PALEO SAUSAGE MEATBALLS

Serv.: 4| **Prep.:** 25m | **Cook:** 6m

Ingredients:
- ✓ 1 apple, chopped
- ✓ 1 onion, chopped
- ✓ 2 tablespoons chopped fresh sage
- ✓ 2 tablespoons chopped fresh rosemary
- ✓ 1/2 teaspoon sea salt
- ✓ 1 pound ground sausage
- ✓ 2 tablespoons olive oil

Directions: In a food processor, mix together the sea salt, rosemary, sage, onion and apple, then pulse until combined well. Add sausage and pulse for 3-4 times until blended.
Roll the sausage mixture into meatballs.
In a big skillet, heat the olive oil on medium heat. Cook the meatballs by batches for 3-4 minutes on each side, with a cover, until it turns brown.

PALEO SEAFOOD CHILI

Serv.: 6| **Prep.:** 20m | **Cook:** 30m

Ingredients:
- ✓ 1 tablespoon olive oil
- ✓ 1 large onion, chopped
- ✓ 1 red bell pepper, chopped
- ✓ 1 green bell pepper, chopped
- ✓ 2 stalks celery, chopped
- ✓ 3 cloves garlic, minced
- ✓ 1 1/2 teaspoons sea salt, divided
- ✓ 1 teaspoon freshly ground pepper, divided
- ✓ 1 (15 ounce) can diced tomatoes
- ✓ 1 cup chicken broth
- ✓ 1 tablespoon dried parsley
- ✓ 2 teaspoons chili powder
- ✓ 3/4 teaspoon cayenne pepper
- ✓ 1 tablespoon tomato paste
- ✓ 1/2 pound sea scallops - rinsed, drained, patted dry, and cut in half
- ✓ 1/2 pound haddock, cut into cubes
- ✓ 1/2 pound uncooked medium shrimp, peeled and deveined

Directions: Heat olive oil at medium-high heat in a large heavy saucepan. Put in garlic, celery, green bell pepper, red bell pepper, and onion; cook until soft, 3 to 4 minutes. Flavor with 1/2 teaspoon of pepper and 1/2 teaspoon of salt. Put in tomatoes and broth; heat to a boil. Lower the heat to medium-low. Put in cayenne pepper, chili powder, and parsley; cook until thickened, for 15 minutes. Blend in tomato paste until dissolved.
Add the remaining 1 teaspoon of salt and 1/2 teaspoon of pepper to flavor the scallop and haddock; add to the saucepan. Mix in shrimp; cook until it is opaque in the center and bright pink on the outside, about 7 minutes.

Let food be thy medicine and medicine be thy food.

- Ippocrate -

CONCLUSION

Thank you again for reading "Paleo Diet for Women"!

I hope you enjoyed reading my book.

Now all you have to do is try making the recipes you like best. You can try to create them as they are listed or make a few small variations in quantities or ingredients.

You will then have the opportunity to experiment with so many recipes for the whole family!

Our health depends on the quality of our food and the PALEO DIET will help you regain energy and health!

I suggest always consulting a nutritionist to figure out which diet is best for you.

Good luck!

Tess Connors

CPSIA information can be obtained
at www.ICGtesting.com
Printed in the USA
BVHW010012180621
609821BV00003B/257

9 781914 561207